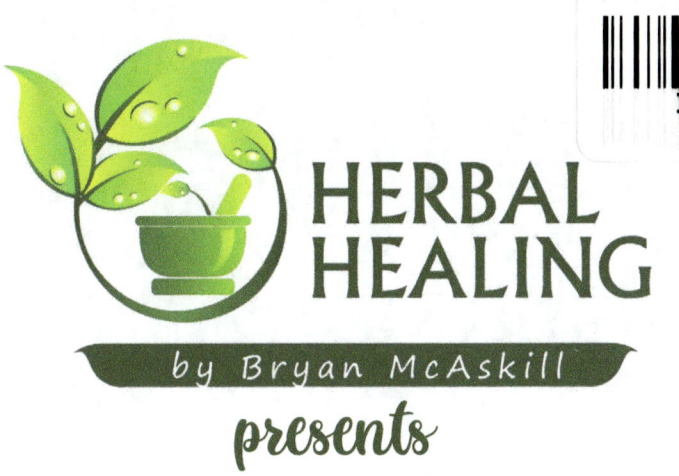

An Alkaline Alphabet:
Coloring Your Way Through The Alphabet

Bryan McAskill

This book is intended to serve as a reference for a healthier lifestyle; not as a medical text. The information provided herein is designed to help readers make informed decisions about their wellness. It is not intended to be a substitute for any specific treatment that may have been prescribed by a doctor. This book is sold with the understanding that the author nor the publisher are not engaged in redering medical advice. If you have a medical condition, it is urged to seek medical help or assistance.

An Alkaline Alphabet introduces babies and toddlers to a colorful variety of alkaline fruits, vegetables, herbs, and spices with pictures for them to easily identify. Teach your child the ABC's and encourage healthy eating habits while reading this book. This book uses pictures of favorite alkaline foods with pronunciations to illustrate each letter of the alphabet from to A-Z.

Also includes lists of benefits for each item, and helpful tips on how to use each food item for parents and caregivers to identify ways they will want to prepare these foods for their child(ren).

Age Range For This Book: Open to all Ages

My intention behind putting this book together is to promote an alkaline and more plant-based lifestyle by introducing children and their parents/guardians to healthier options. Our children are often persuaded into craving unnatural snacks, foods, and drinks filled with chemicals and ingredients that are detrimental to the human body.

Children can recognize most of the unhealthy foods but are far too often presented with only drawings or cartoon-like images when it comes to healthier foods. I have made the effort of also providing real-life images of each item in this book to take a step away from the cartoon-like images children are presented with when viewing healthier options so they can become more easily recognizable to children and readers of this book.

Use this book to teach the alphabet and pronunciation, while learning about healthier options, and getting creative with using ingredients however you see fit.

About the author:

Bryan McAskill is an Herbalist, Outpatient Clinician, Coach, and Naturopathic Alternative-Health educator from Lynn, MA (USA) who teaches holistic wellness through Alkaline, plant-based modalities. He is passionate about providing nutrition information and healthy food options to communities.

How to Read the text in this Book

name of each item

how to pronounce item

Blackberries
(blak•beh•reez)

high in fiber, boosts brain health, improves memory and bone health

health benefits of each item

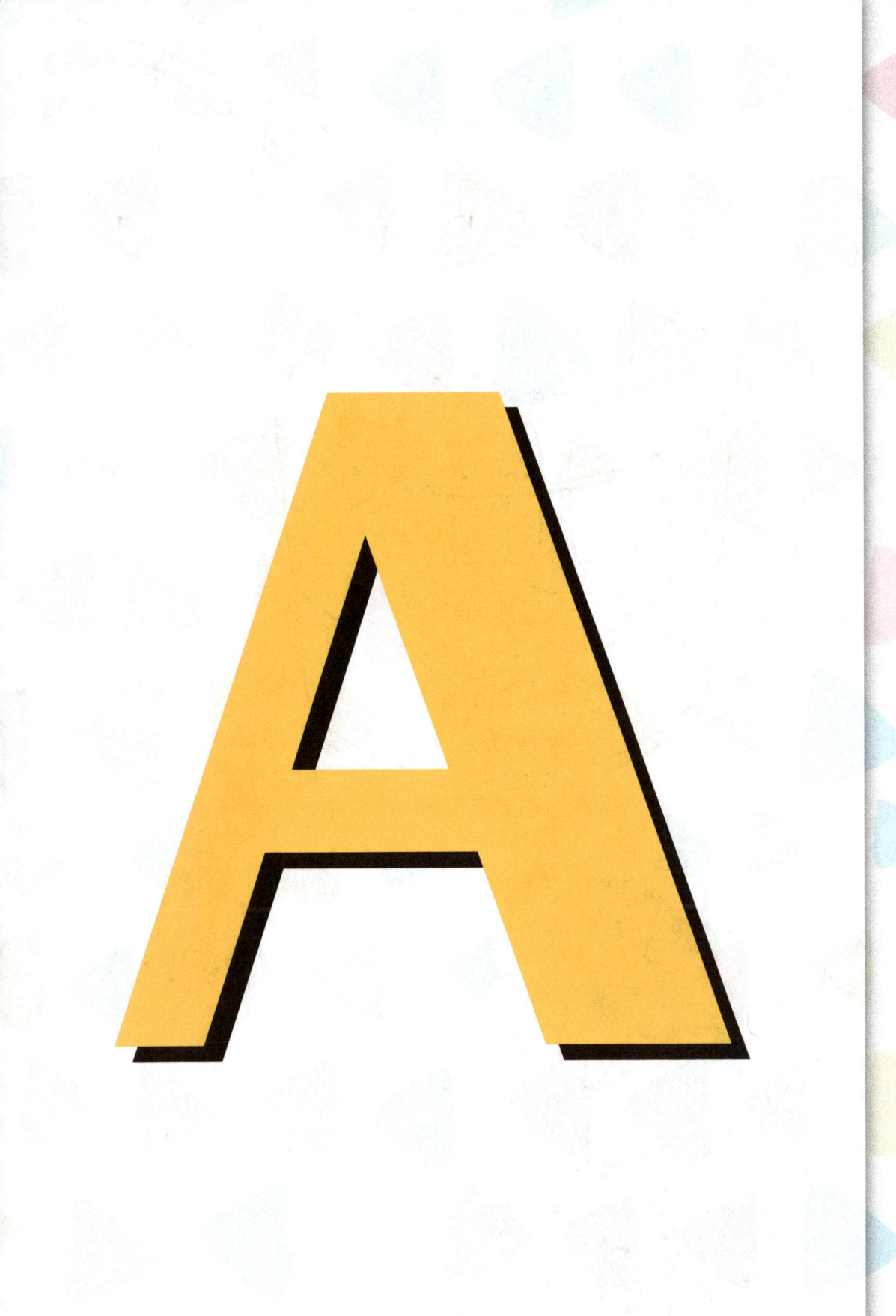

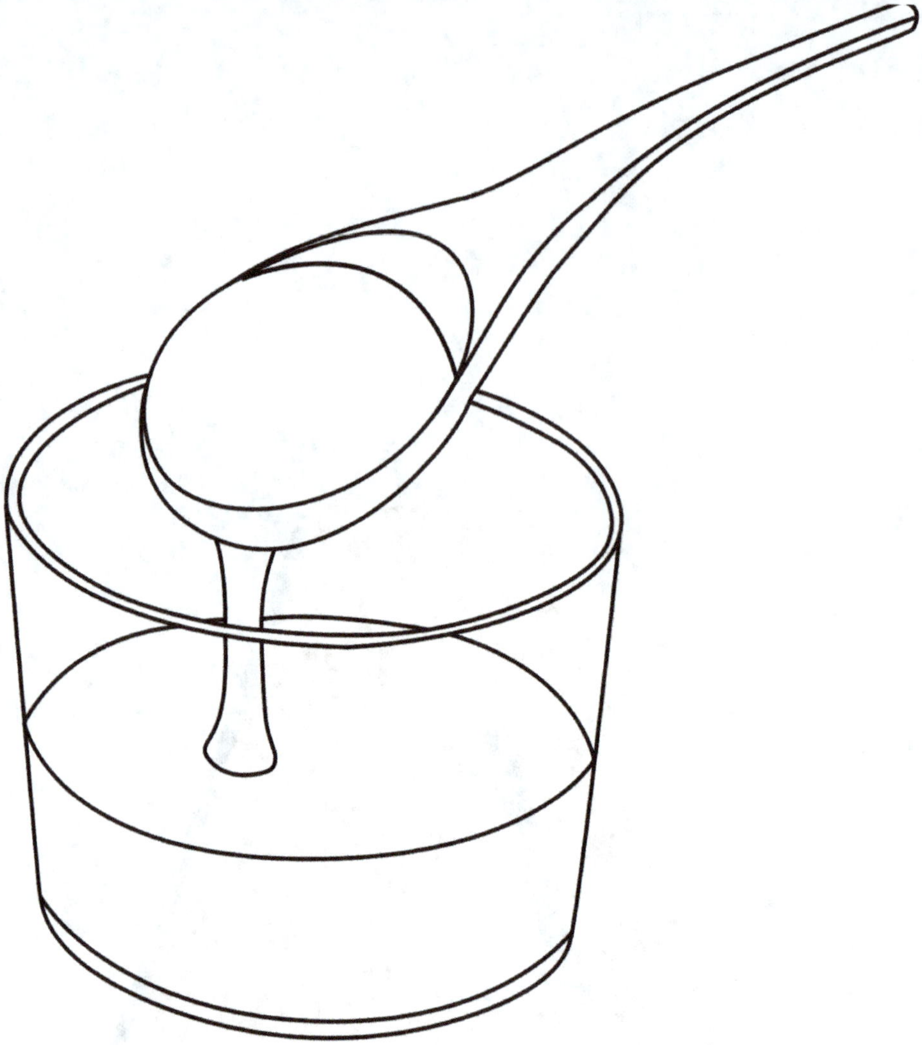

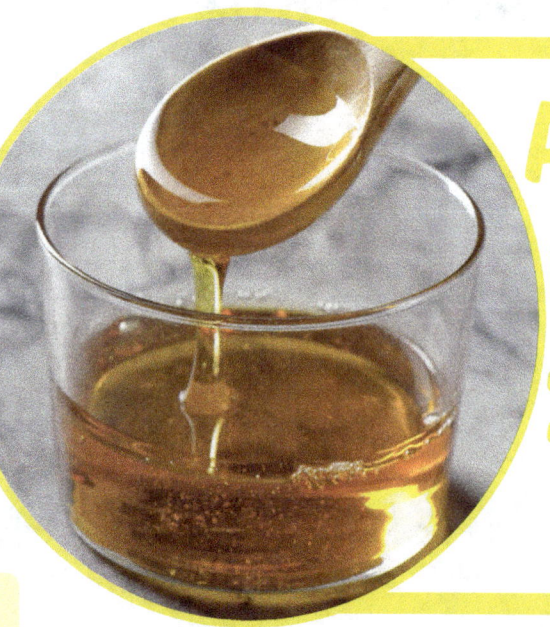

Agave (Nectar)
(uh•gaa•vei)

control blood sugar, lowers cholesterol, helps metabolism

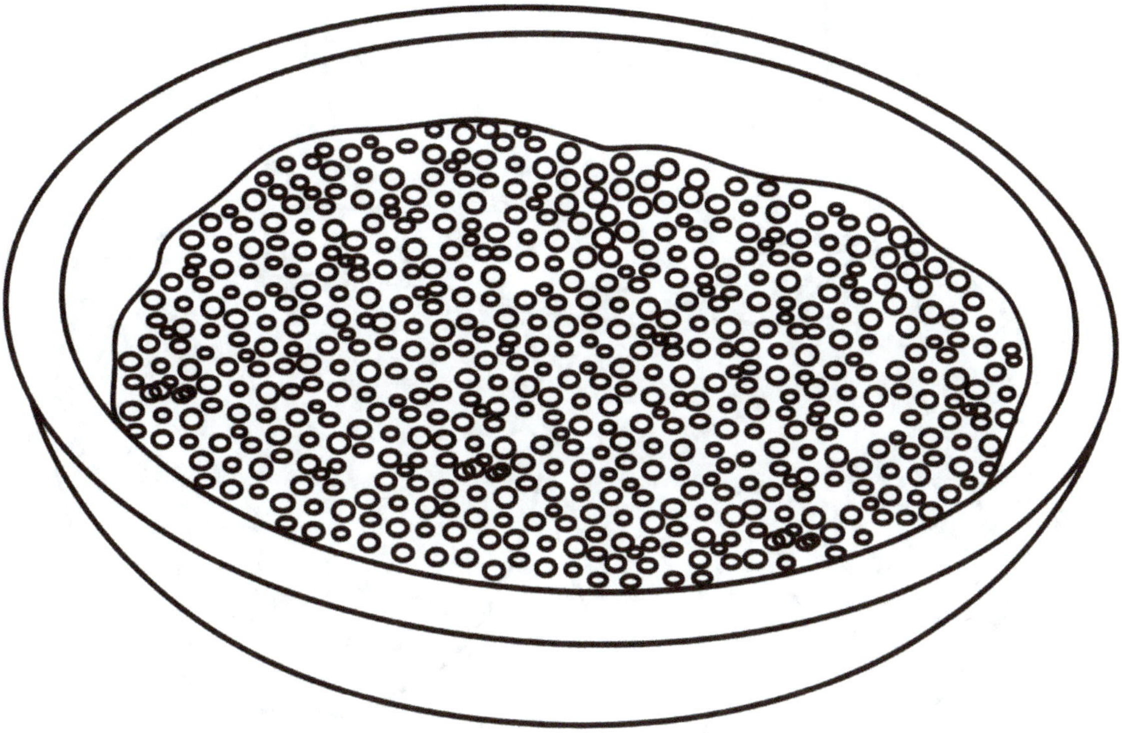

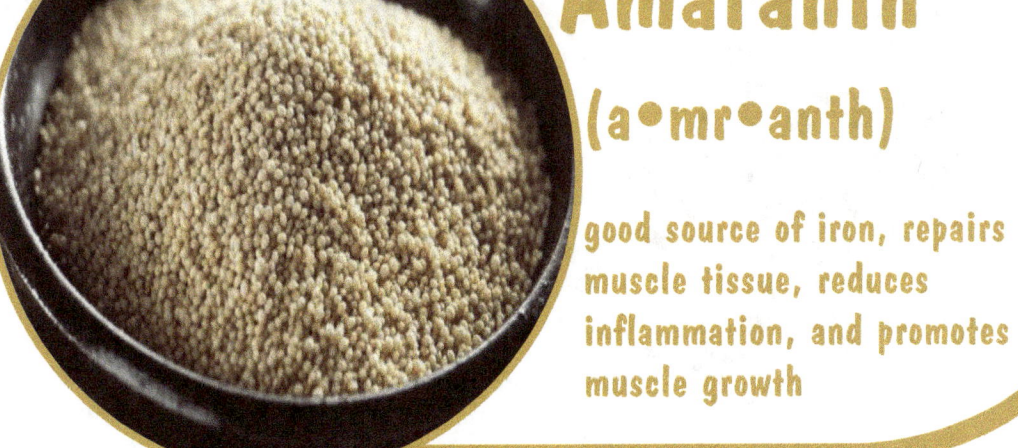

Amaranth
(a•mr•anth)

good source of iron, repairs muscle tissue, reduces inflammation, and promotes muscle growth

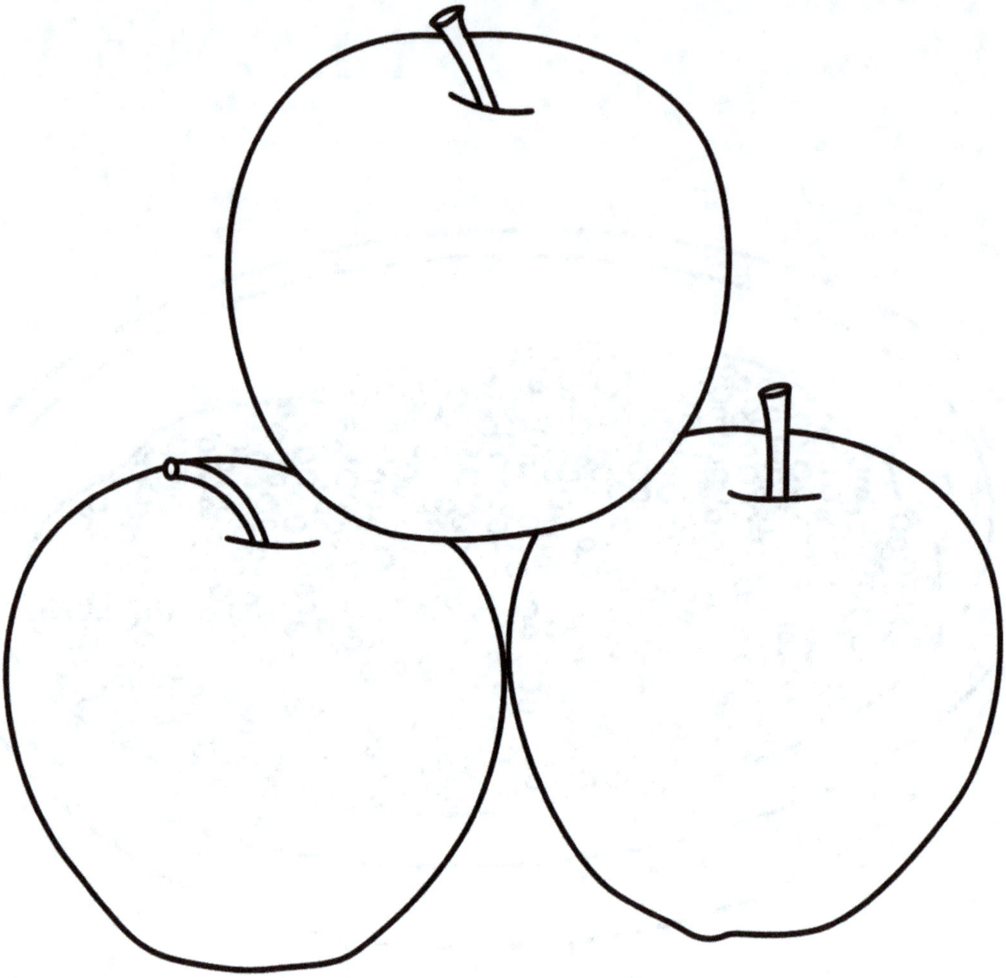

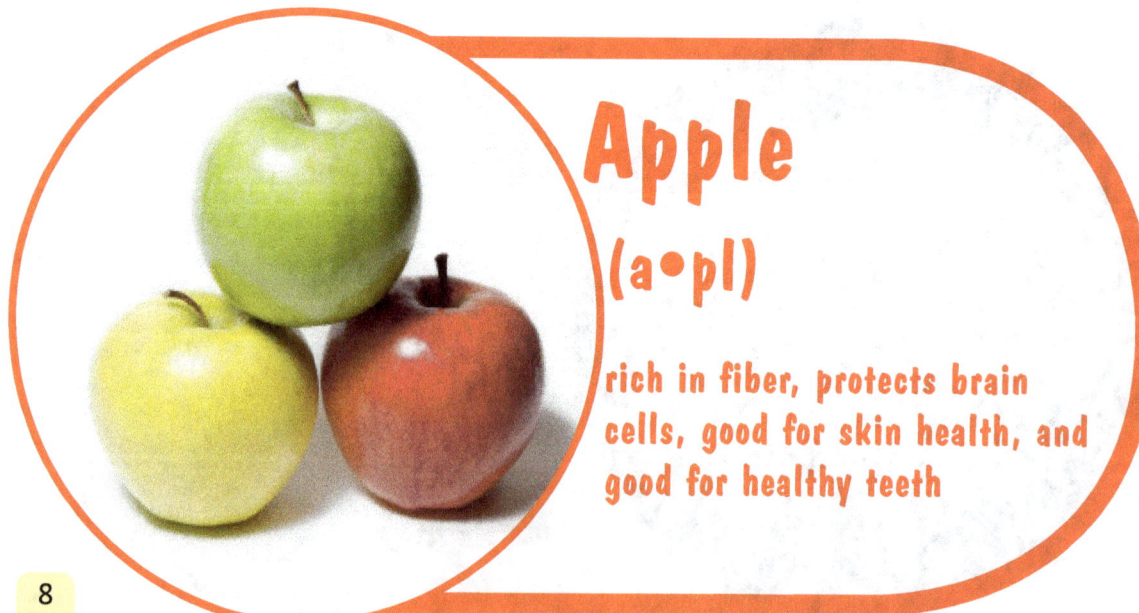

Apple
(a•pl)

rich in fiber, protects brain cells, good for skin health, and good for healthy teeth

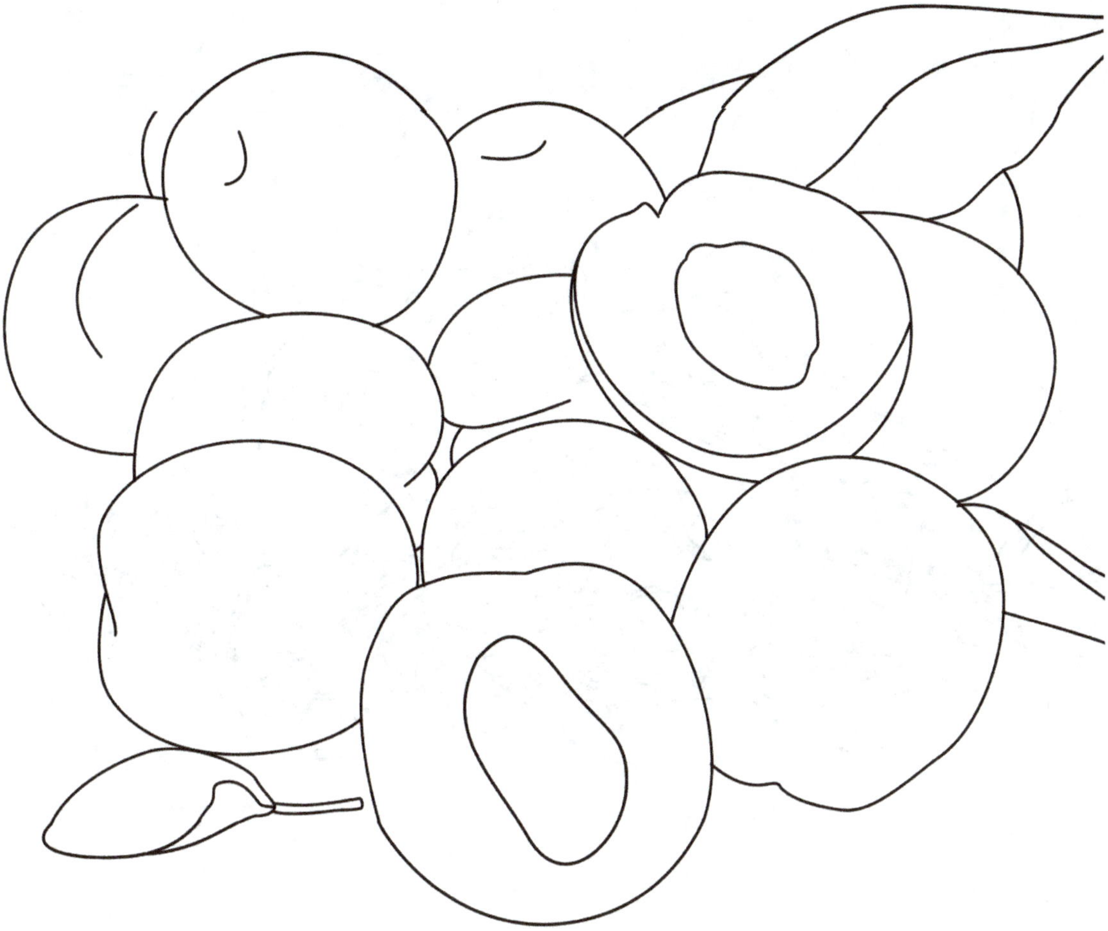

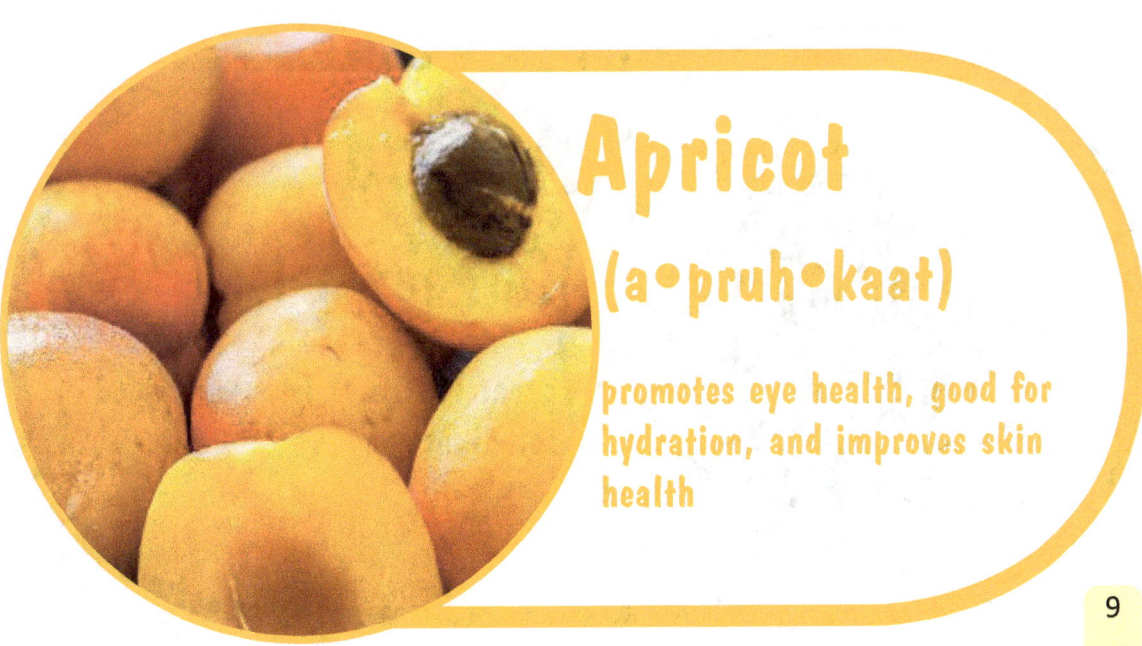

Apricot
(a•pruh•kaat)

promotes eye health, good for hydration, and improves skin health

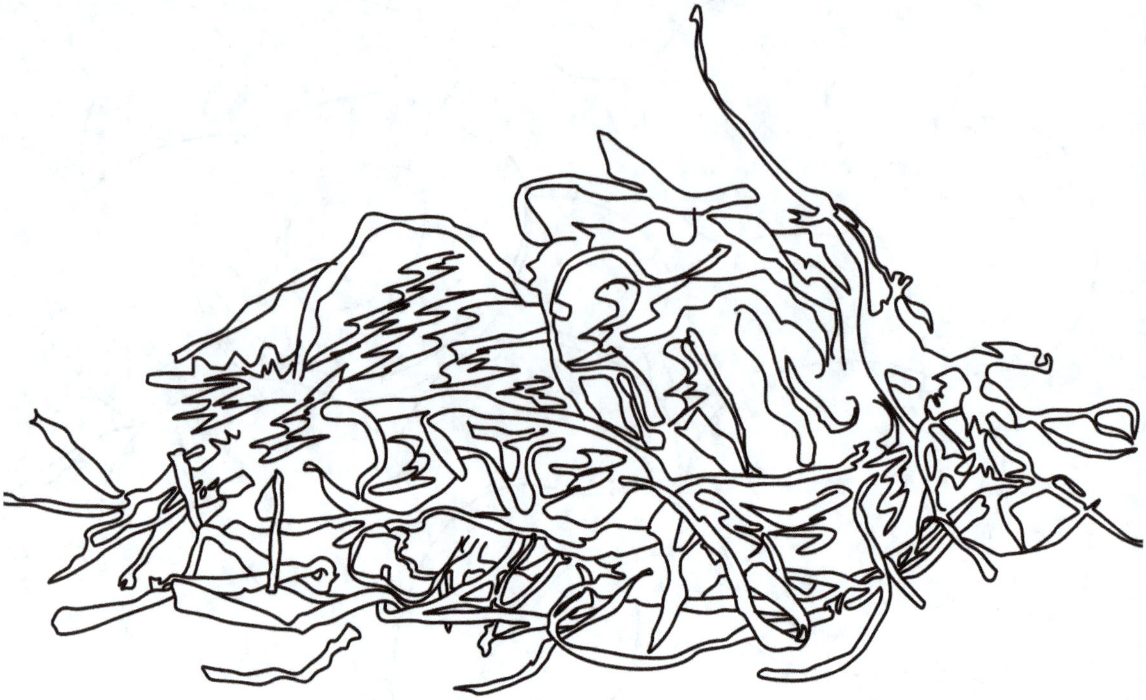

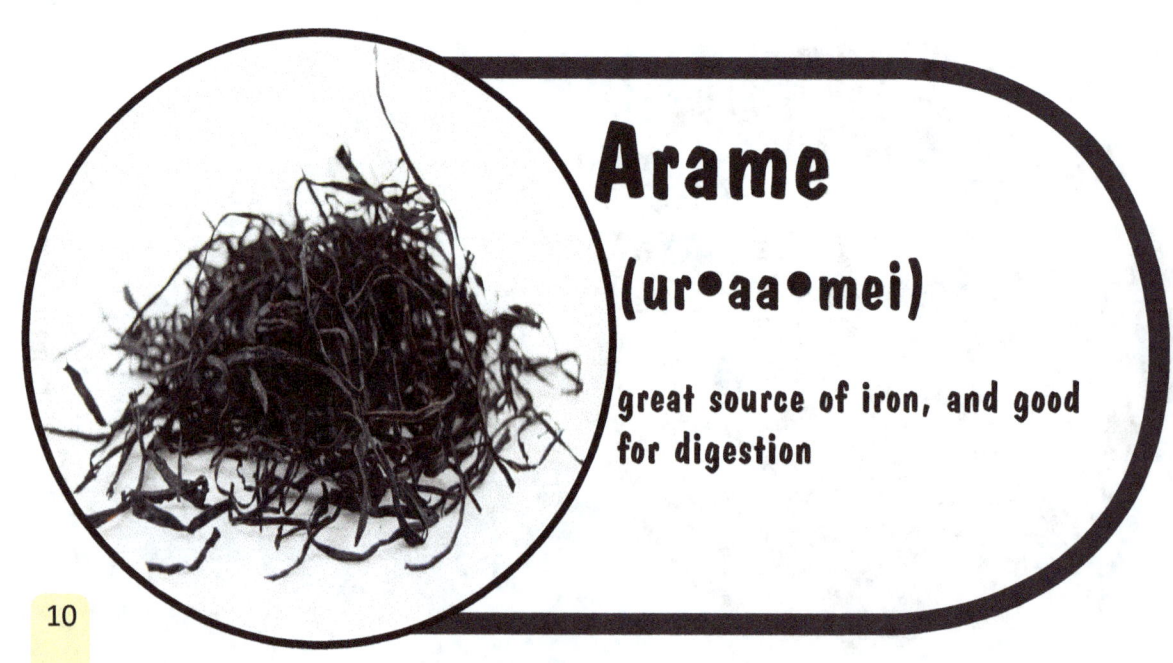

Arame

(ur•aa•mei)

great source of iron, and good for digestion

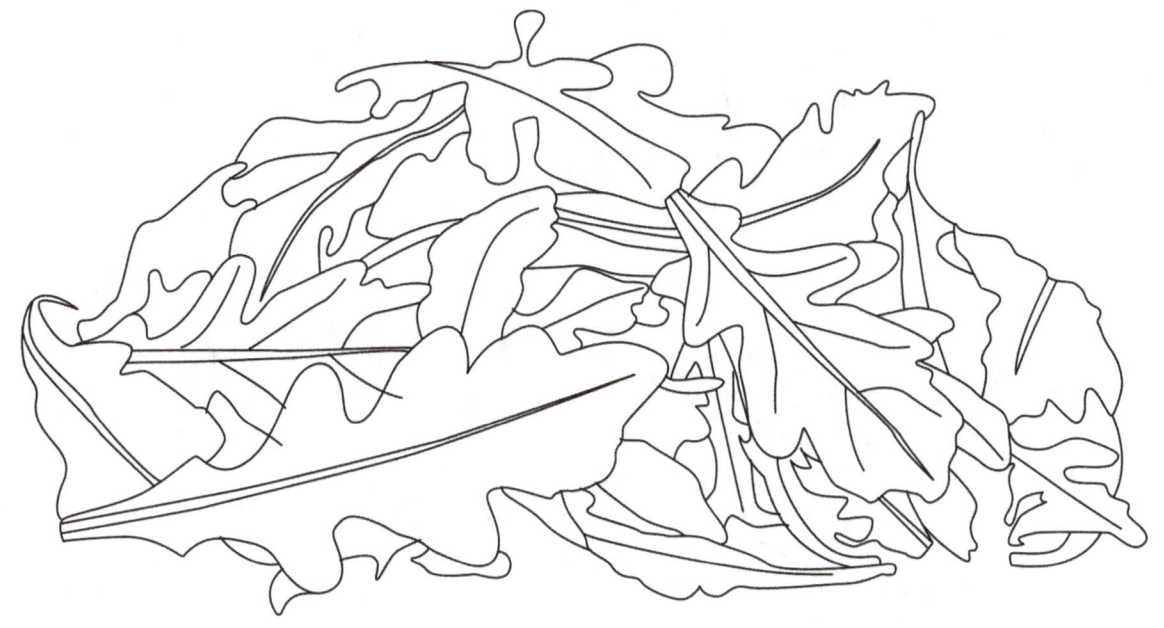

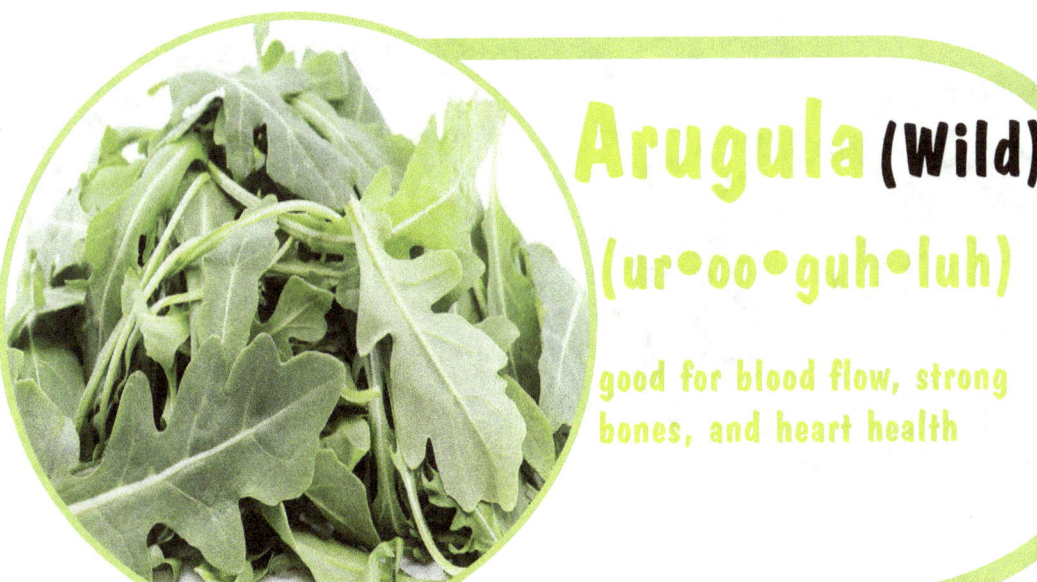

Arugula (Wild)

(ur•oo•guh•luh)

good for blood flow, strong bones, and heart health

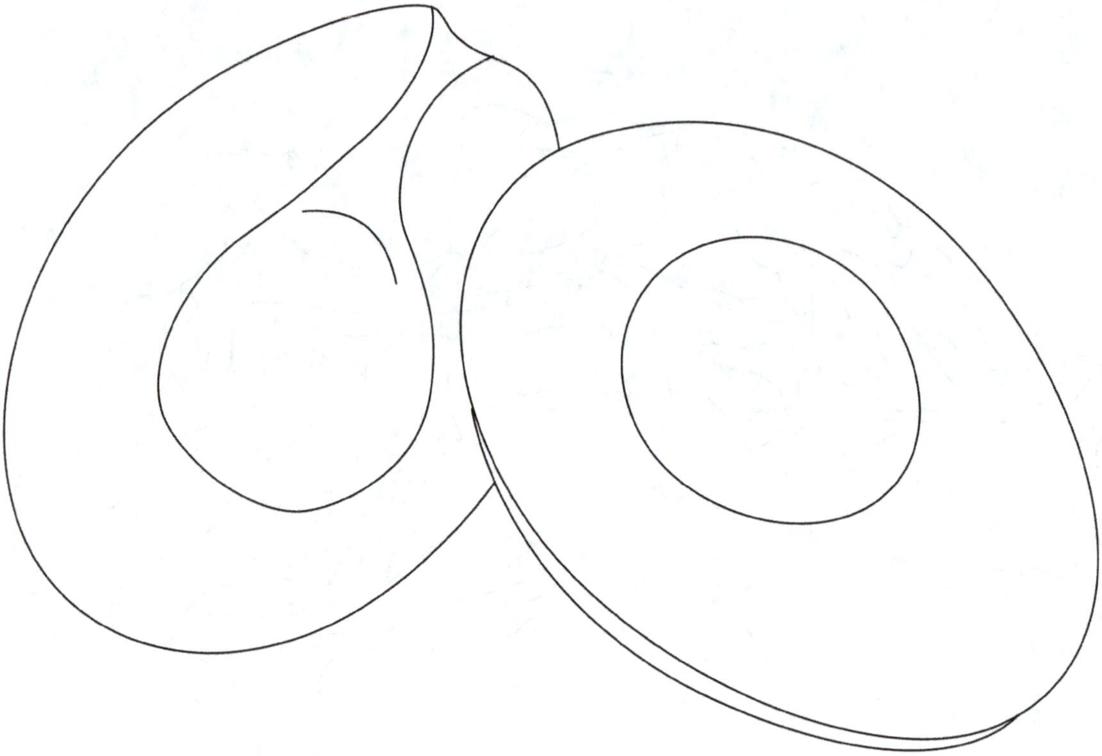

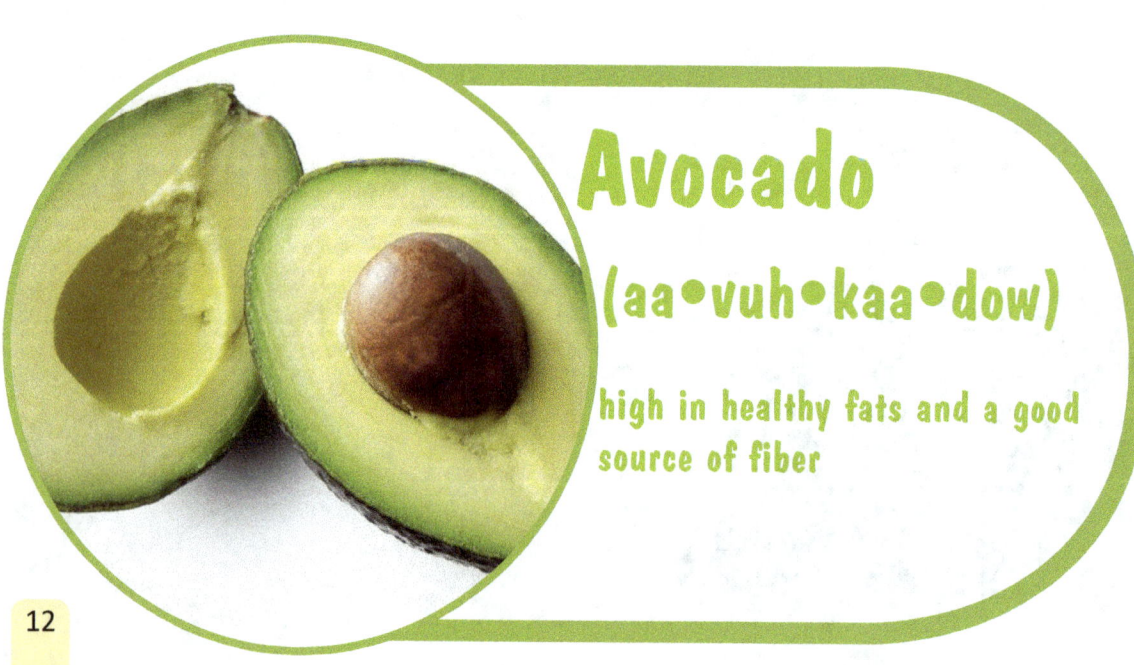

Avocado
(aa•vuh•kaa•dow)

high in healthy fats and a good source of fiber

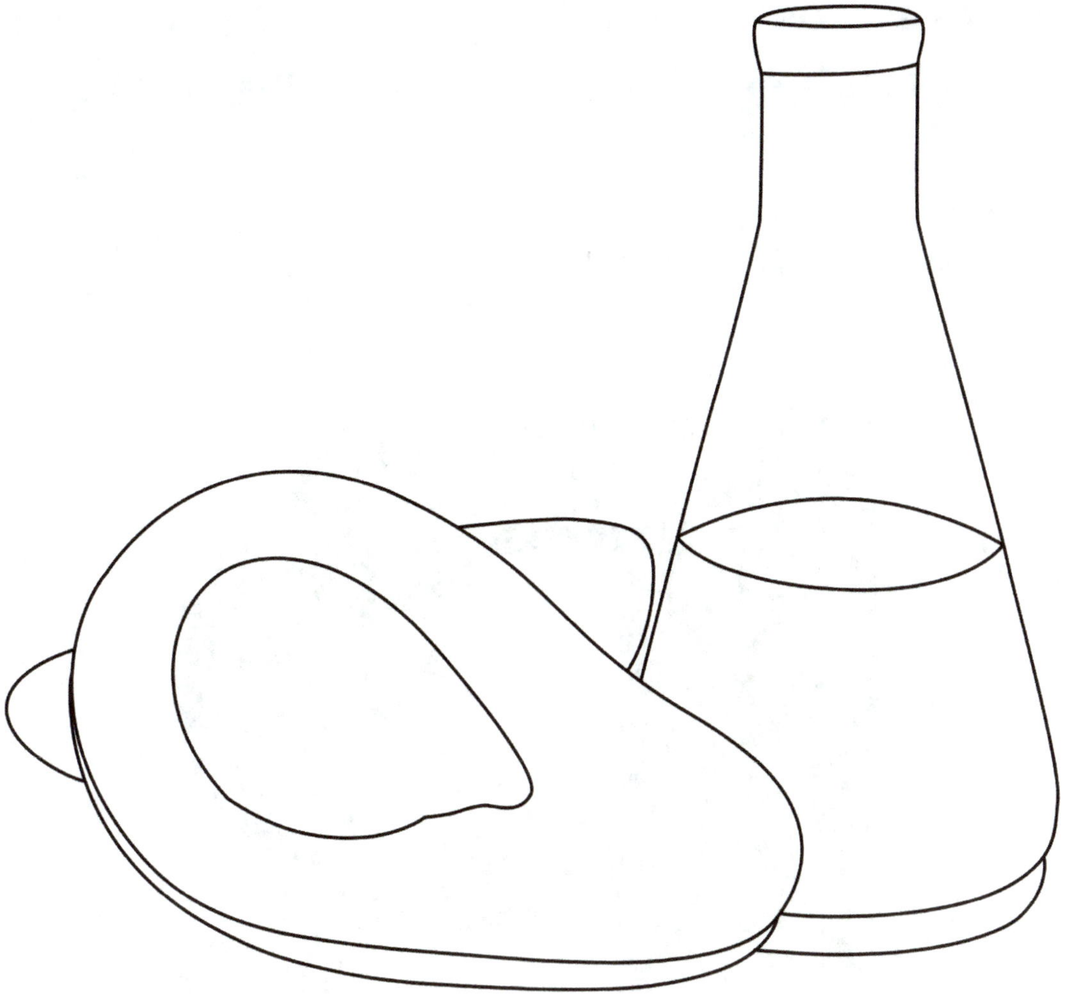

Avocado Oil
(aa•vuh•kaa•dow oyl)

abundant in healthy fatty acids, improves heart health, balances cholesterol, good for hair, skin and nails)

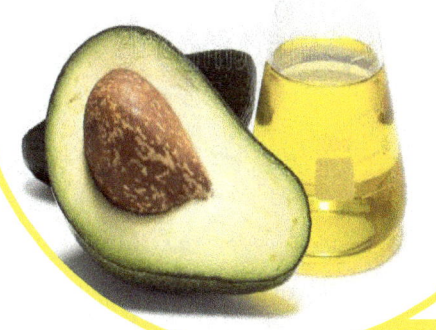

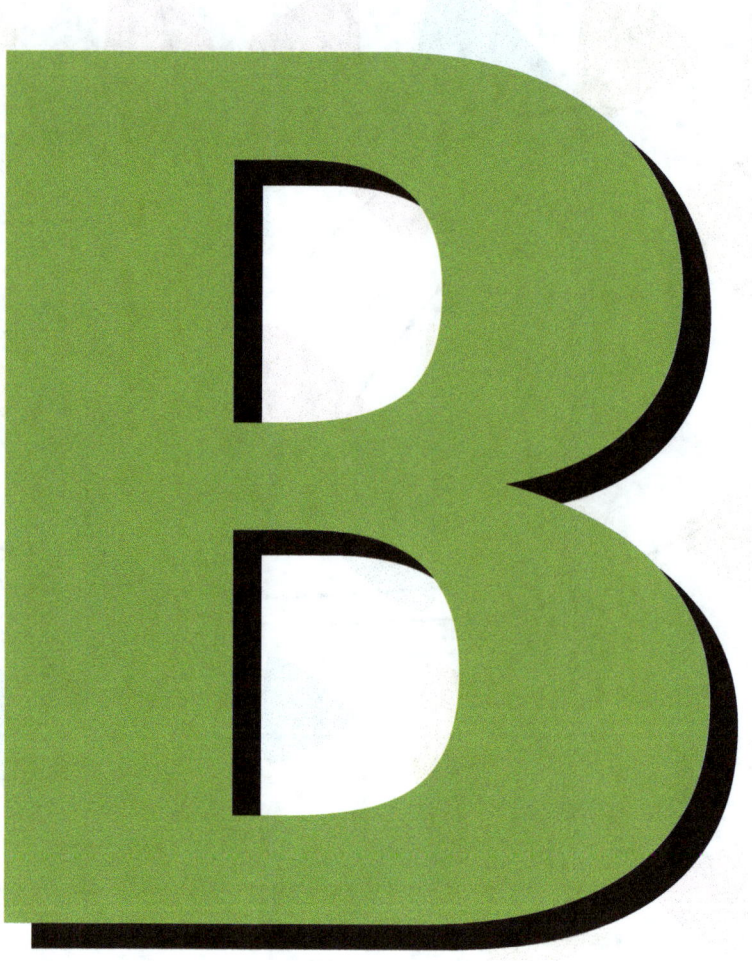

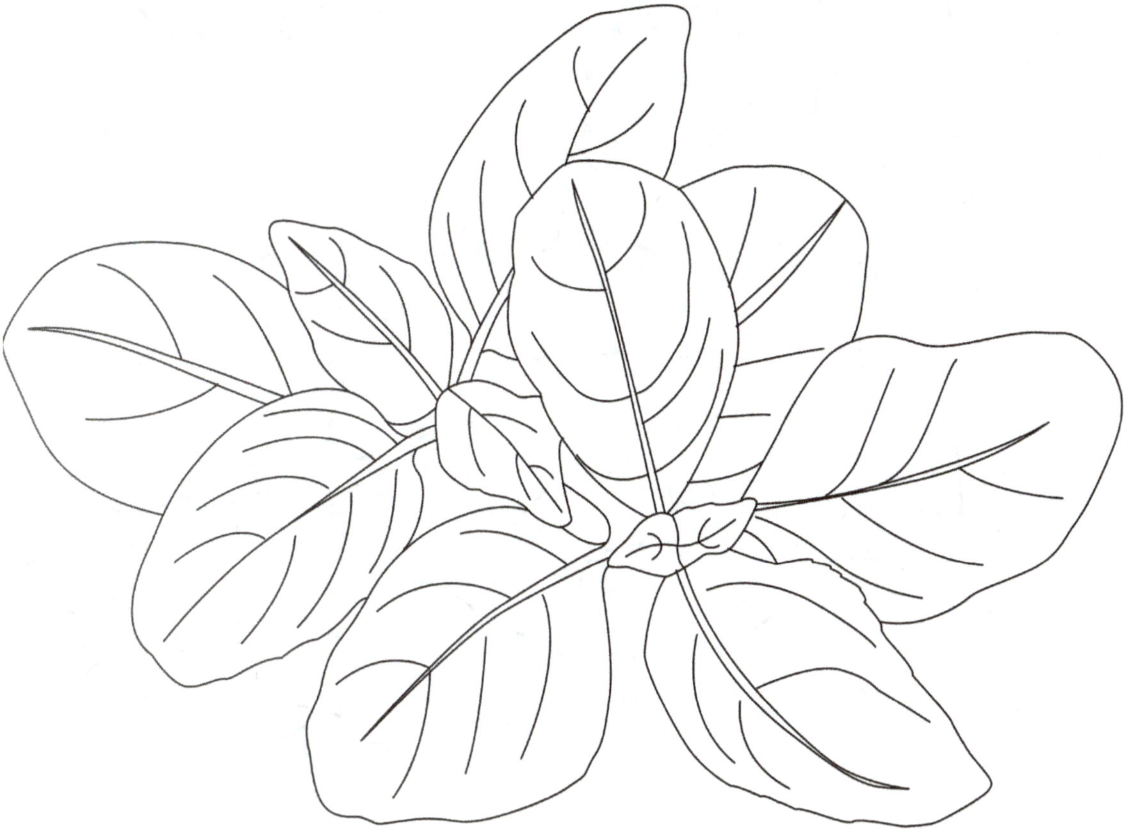

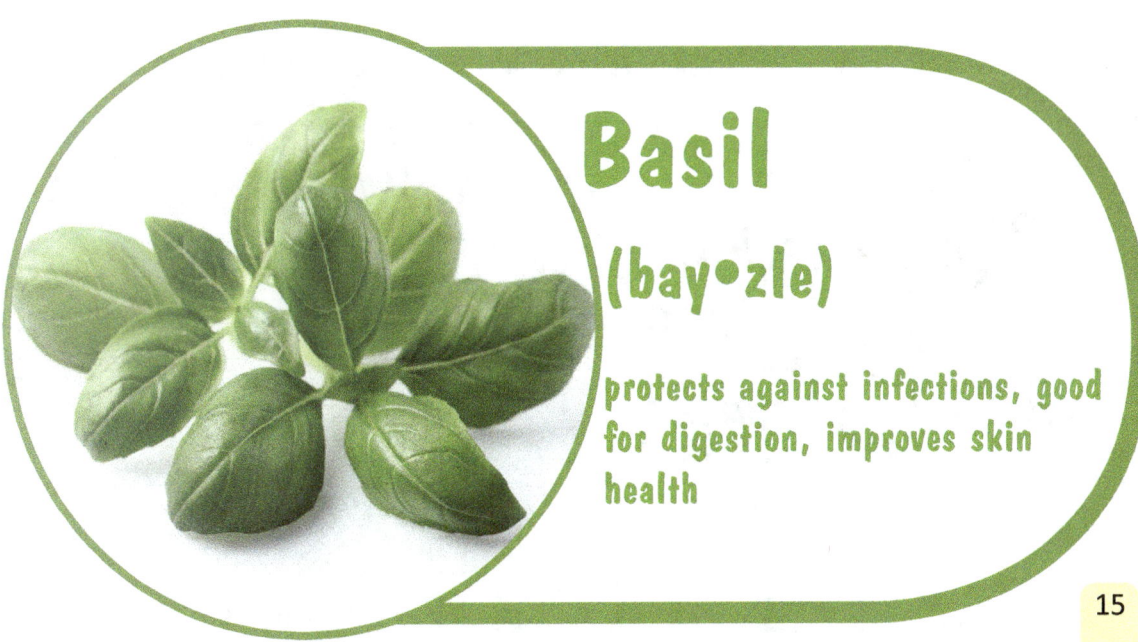

Basil

(bay•zle)

protects against infections, good for digestion, improves skin health

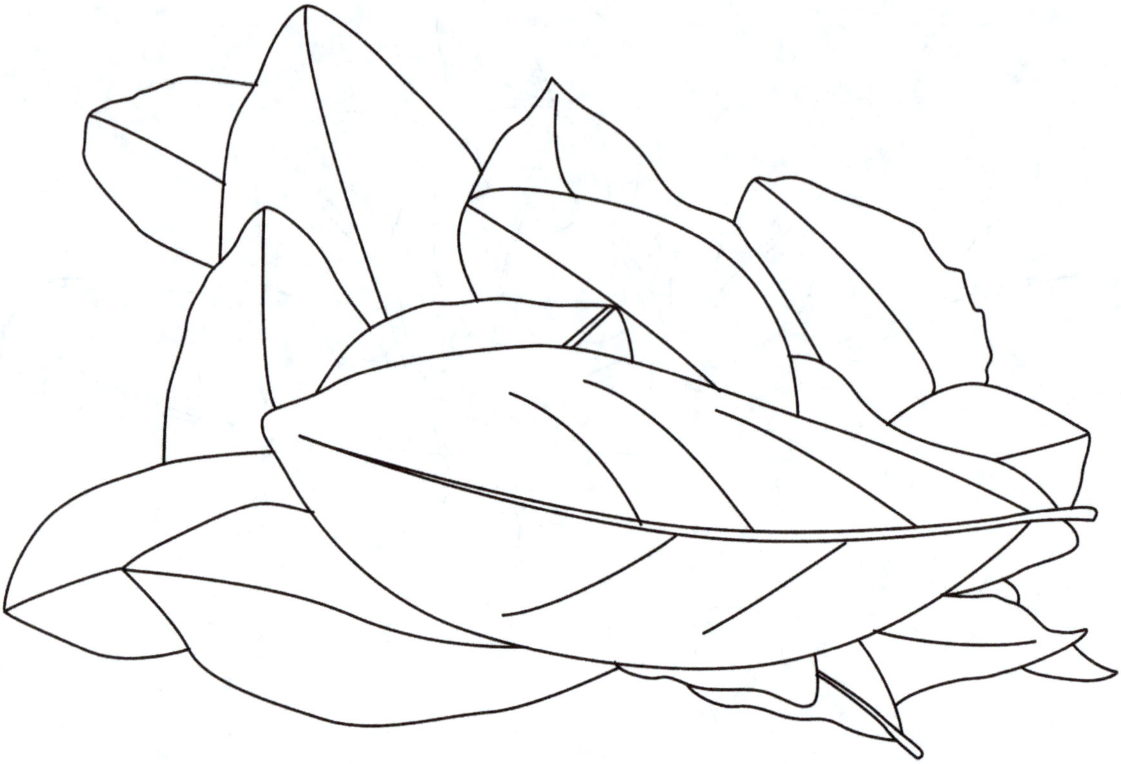

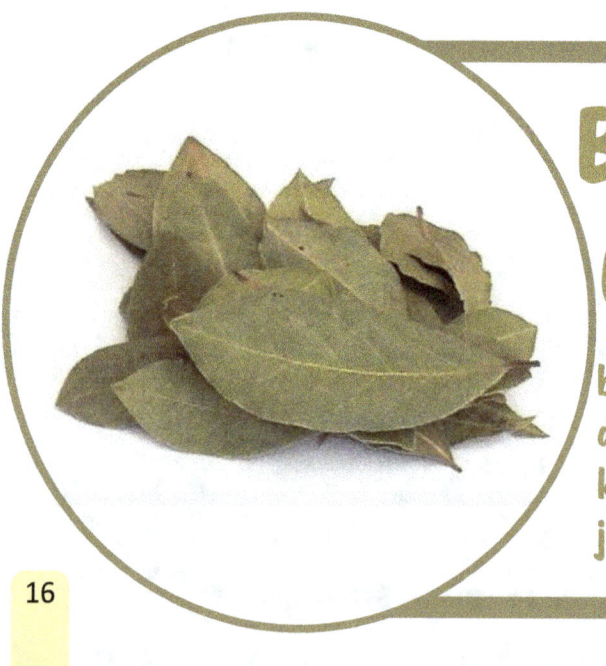

Bay Leaf
(bei leef)

builds strong immune system, digestion health, good for the kidneys and treating bone and joint pain

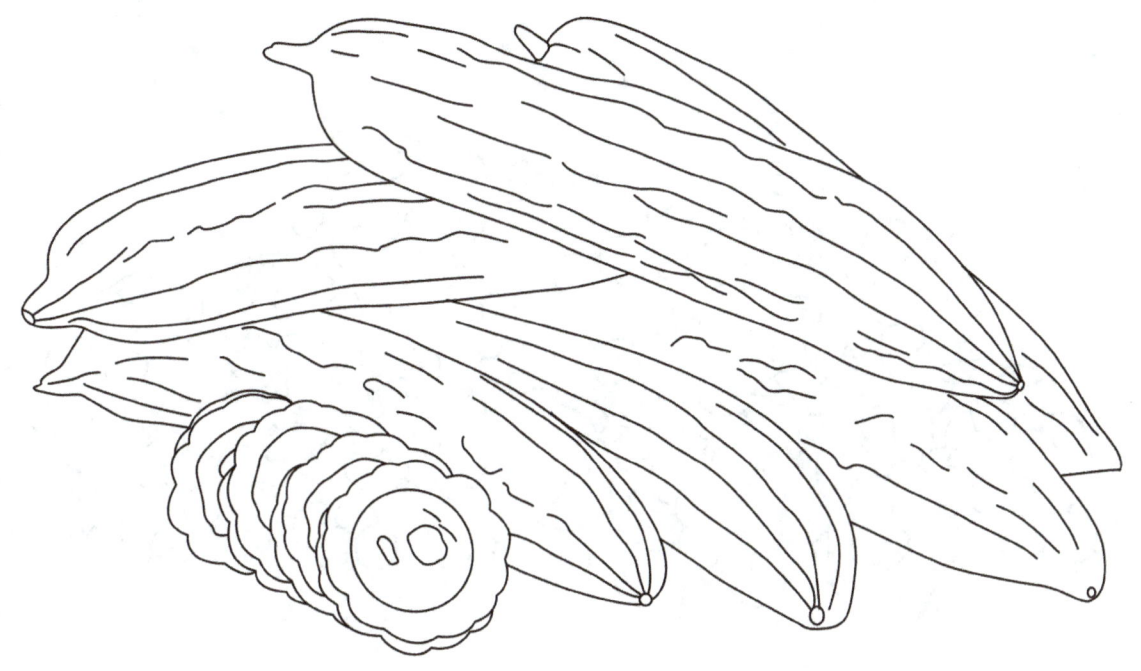

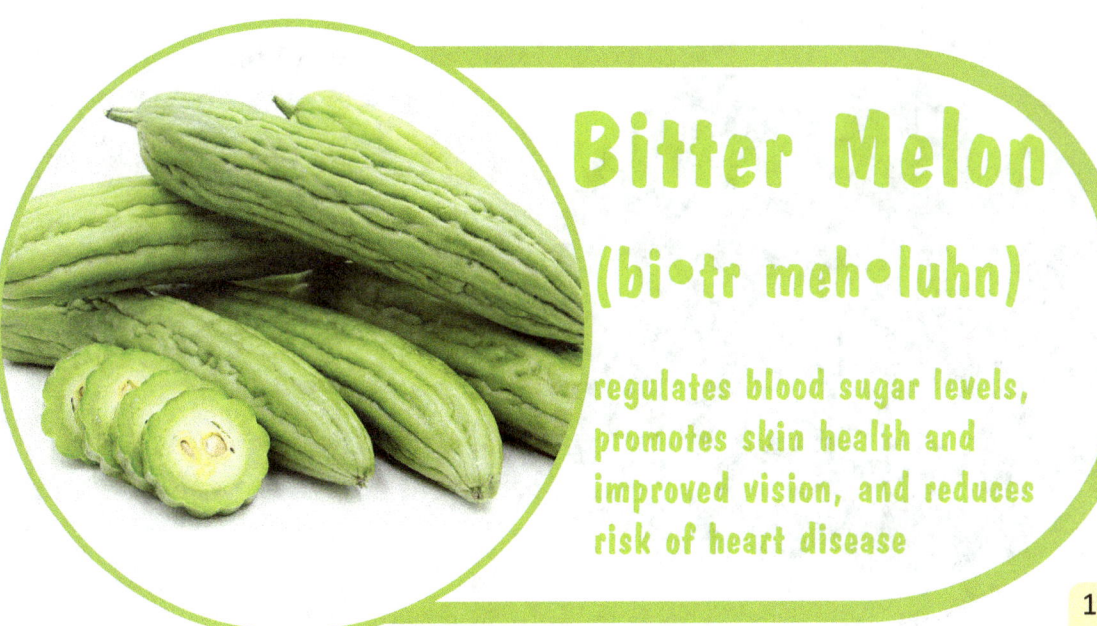

Bitter Melon
(bi•tr meh•luhn)

regulates blood sugar levels, promotes skin health and improved vision, and reduces risk of heart disease

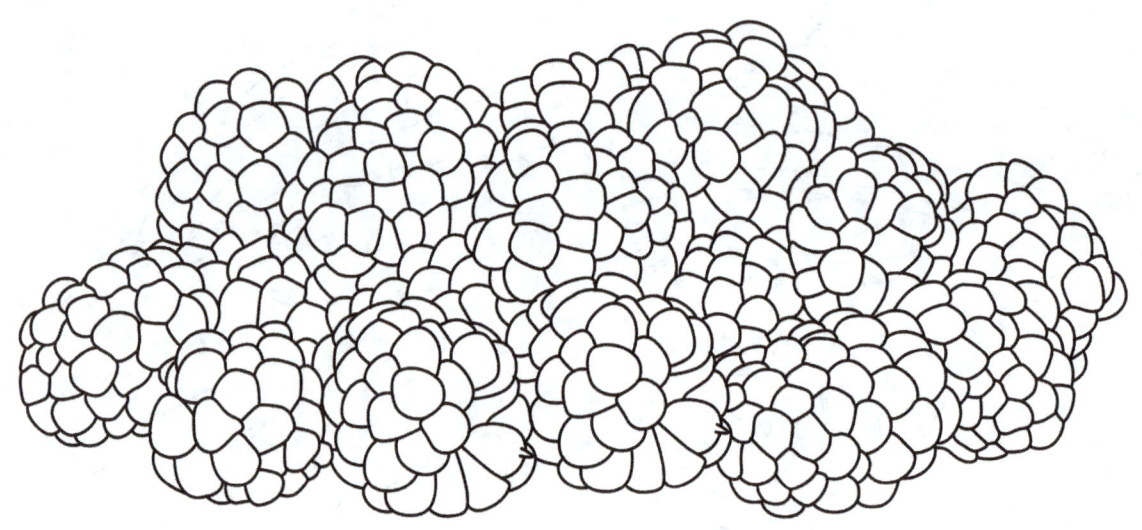

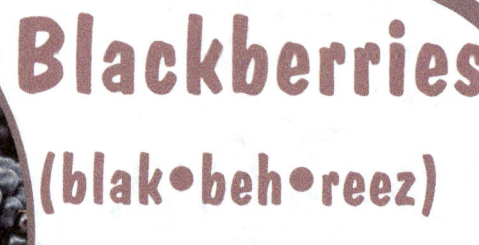

Blackberries
(blak•beh•reez)

high in fiber, boosts brain health, improves memory and bone health

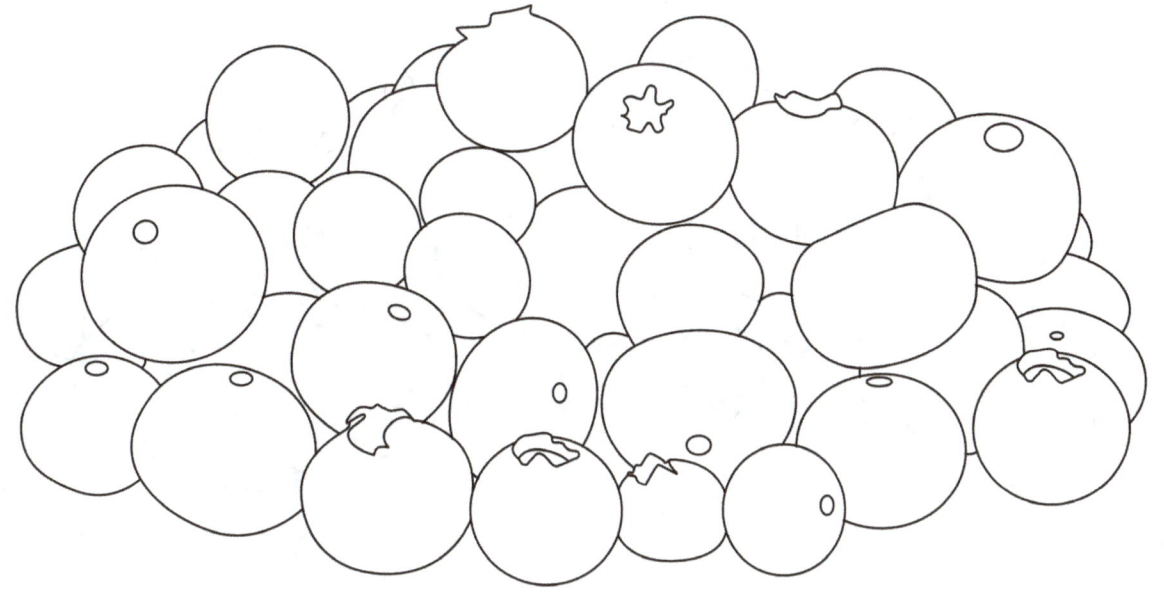

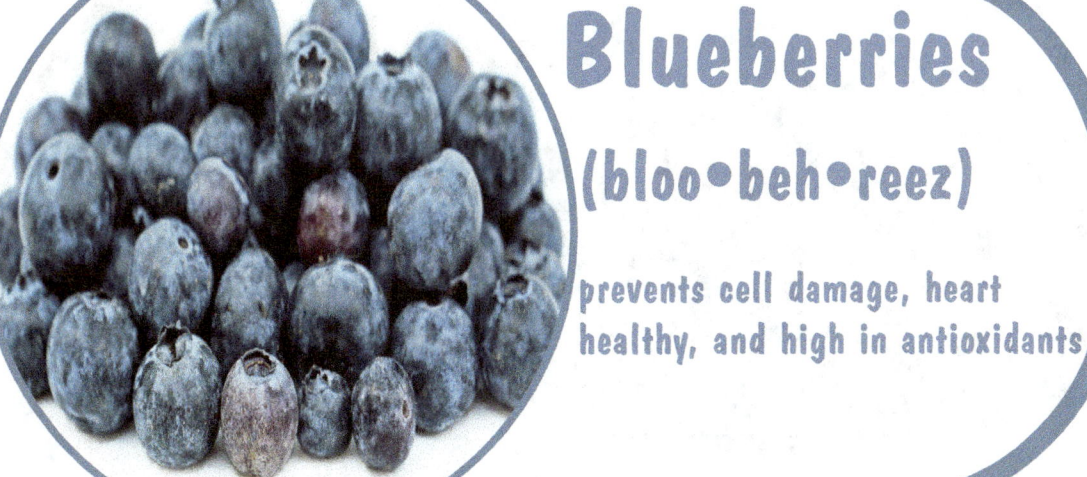

Blueberries
(bloo•beh•reez)

prevents cell damage, heart healthy, and high in antioxidants

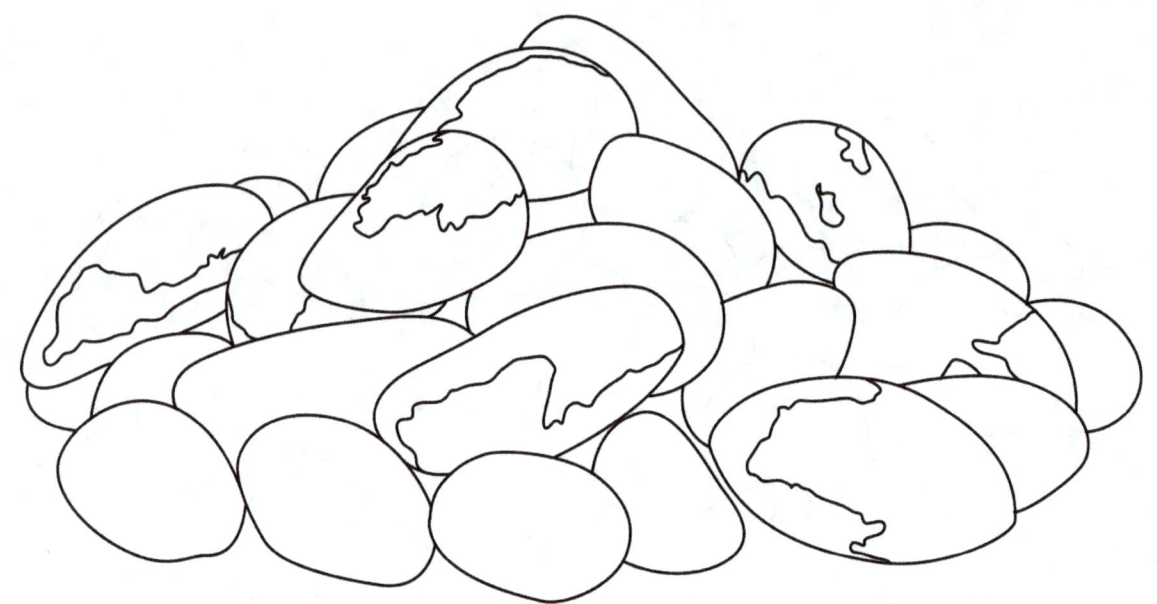

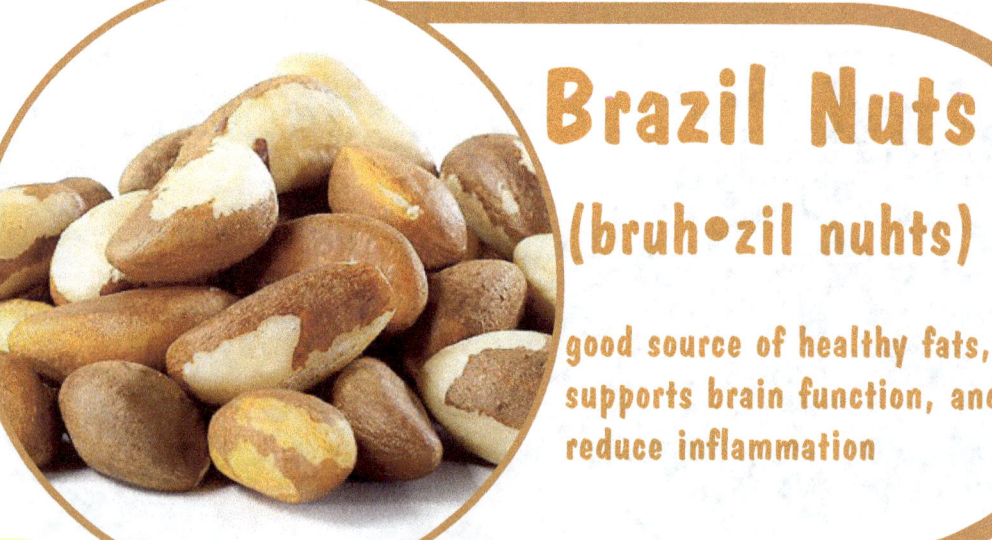

Brazil Nuts
(bruh•zil nuhts)

good source of healthy fats, supports brain function, and reduce inflammation

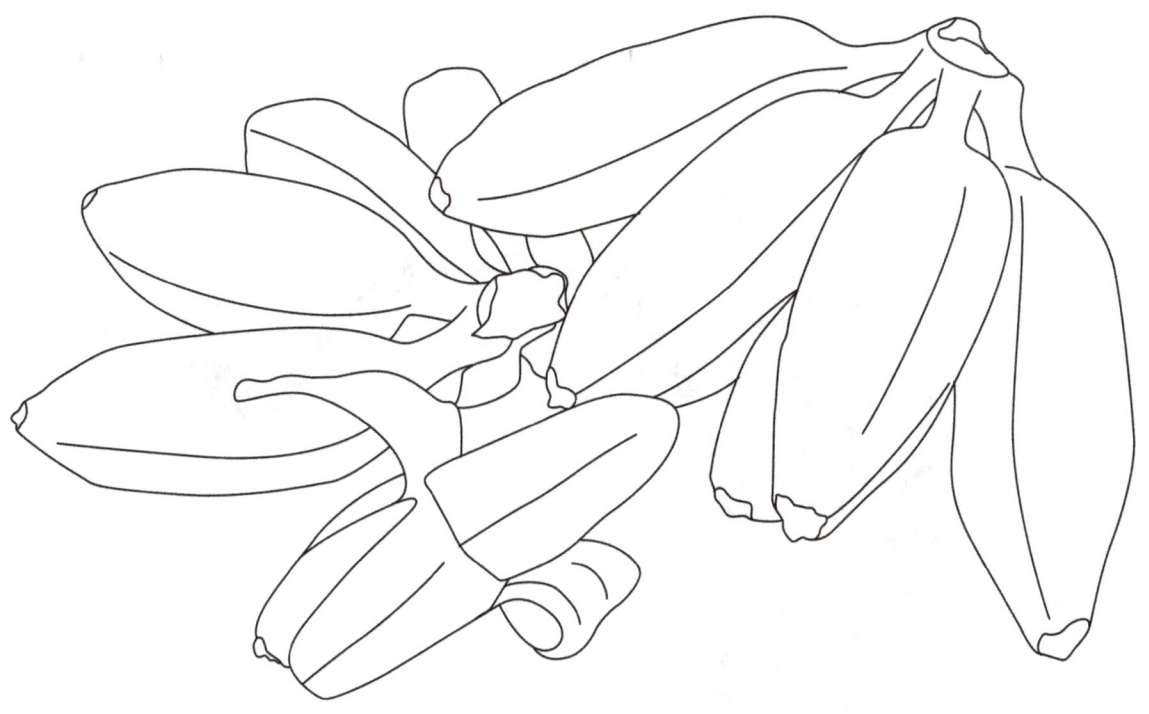

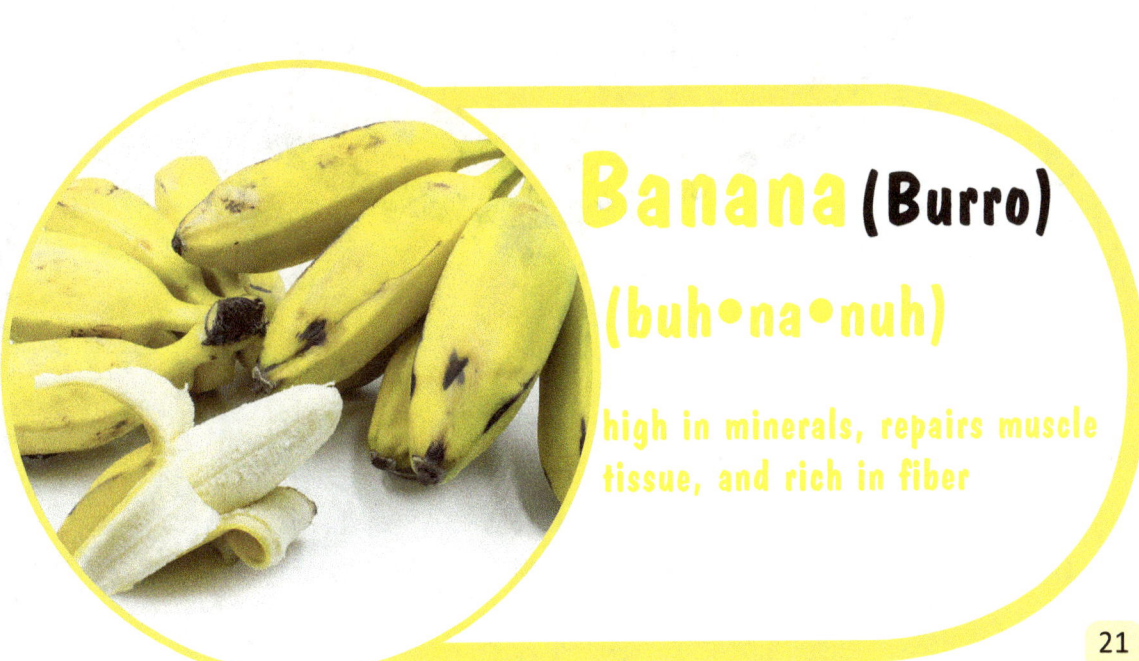

Banana (Burro)
(buh•na•nuh)

high in minerals, repairs muscle tissue, and rich in fiber

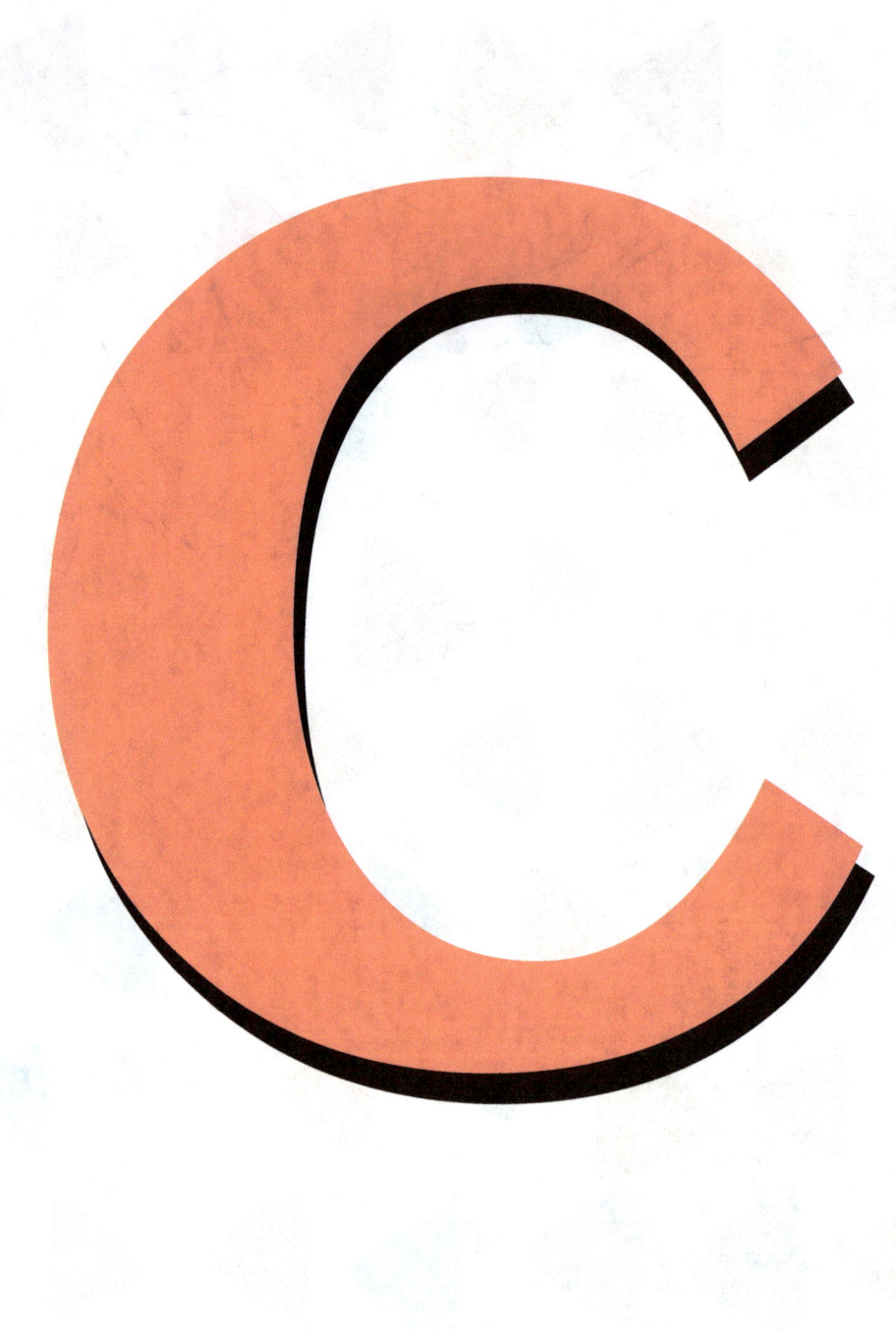

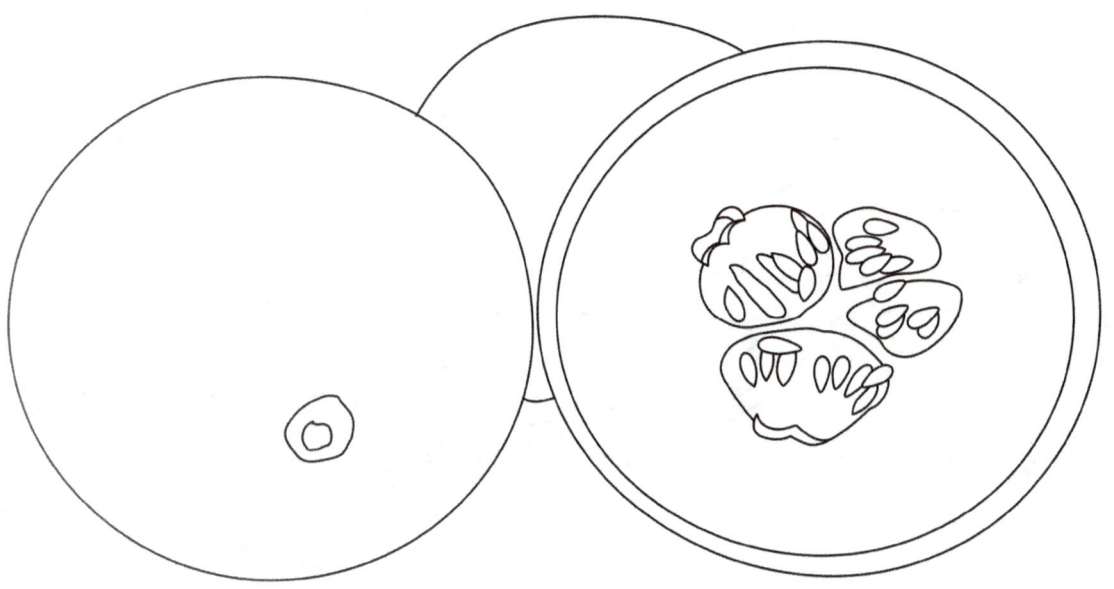

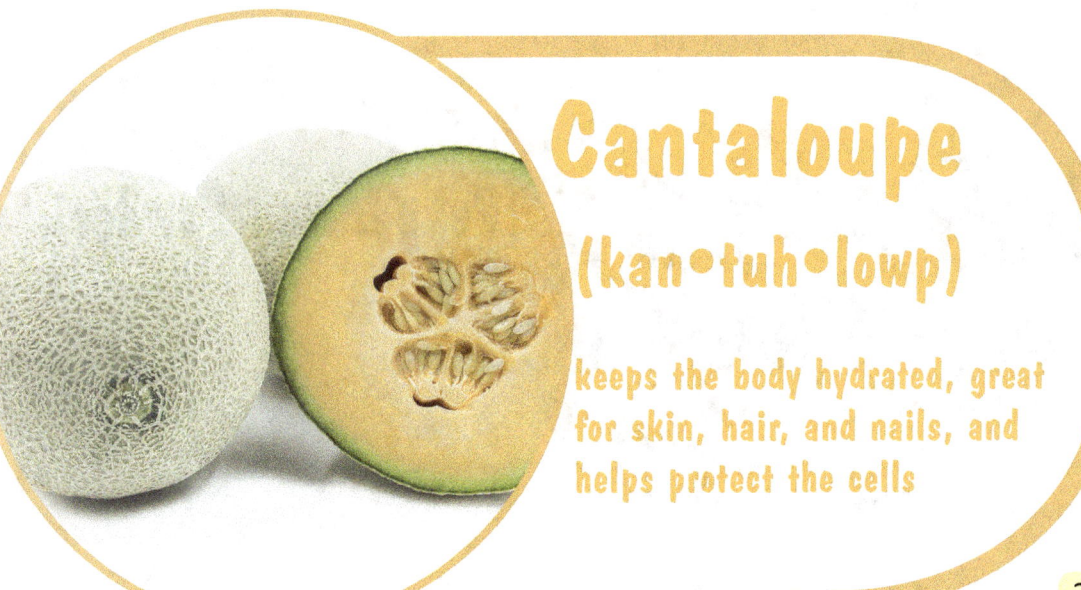

Cantaloupe
(kan•tuh•lowp)

keeps the body hydrated, great for skin, hair, and nails, and helps protect the cells

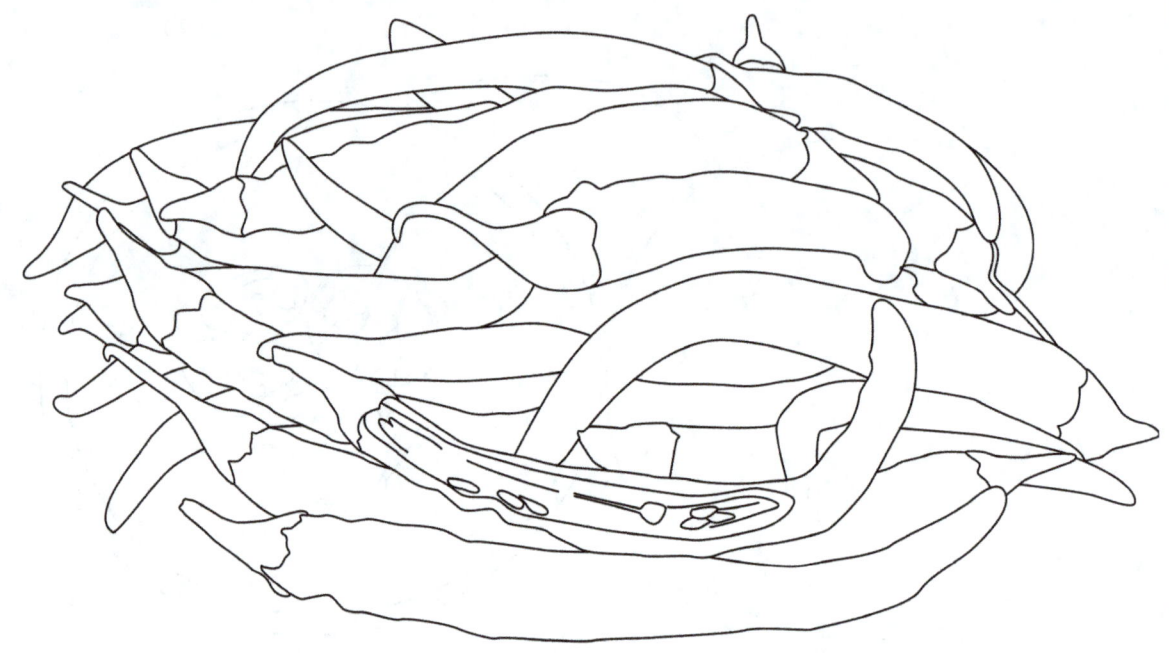

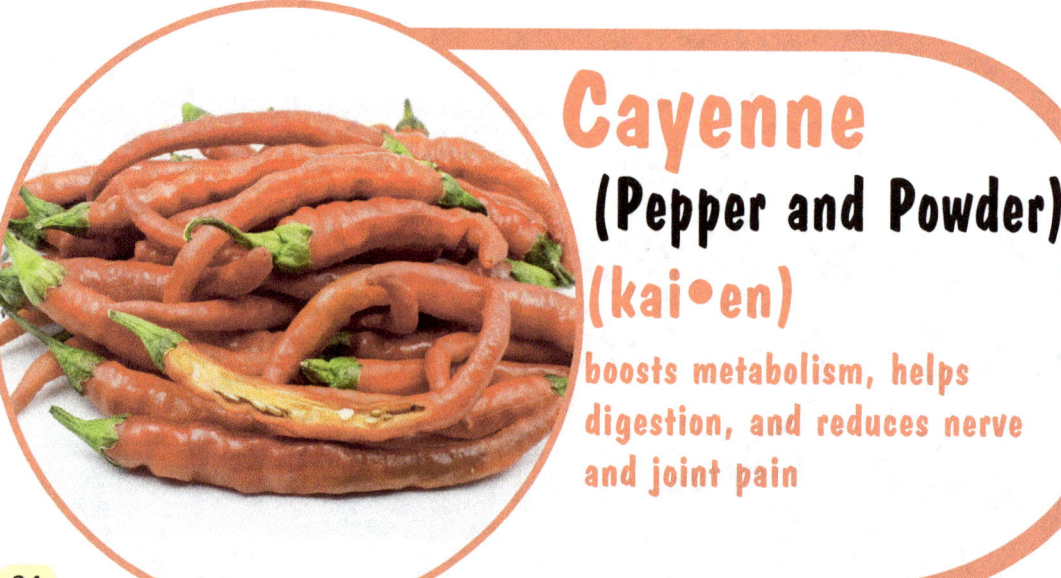

Cayenne
(Pepper and Powder)
(kai•en)

boosts metabolism, helps digestion, and reduces nerve and joint pain

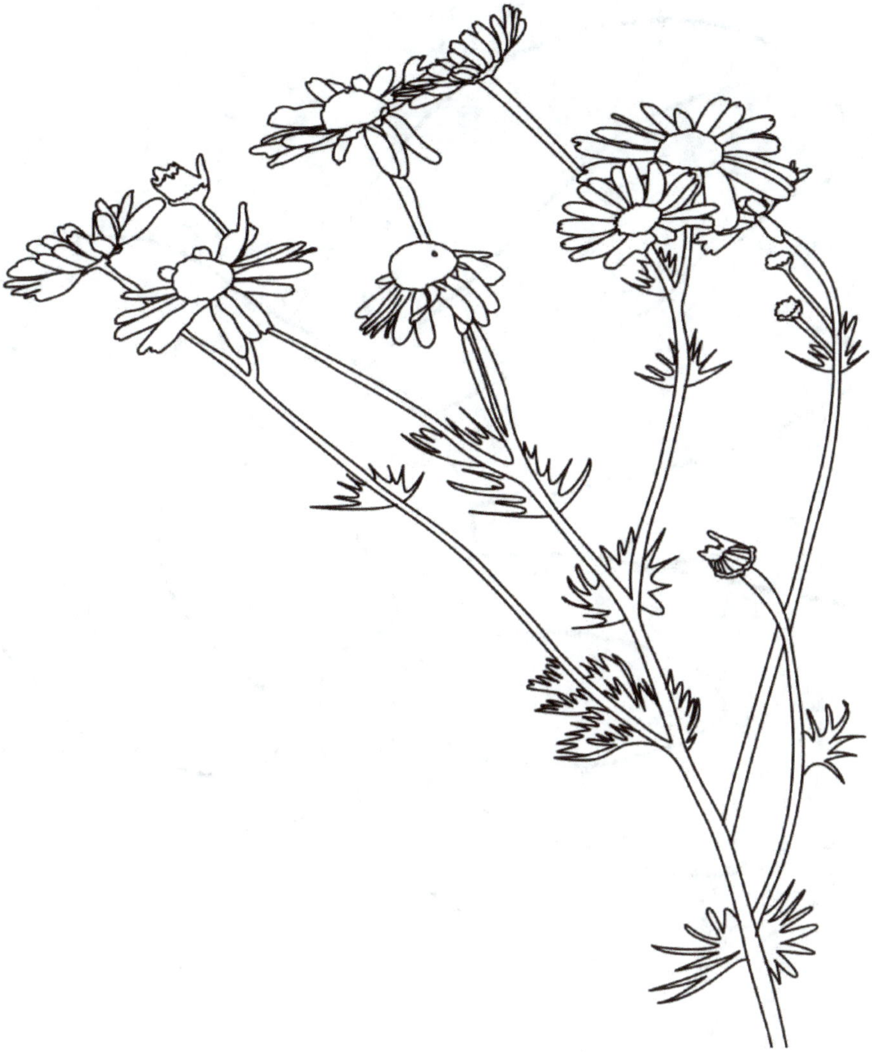

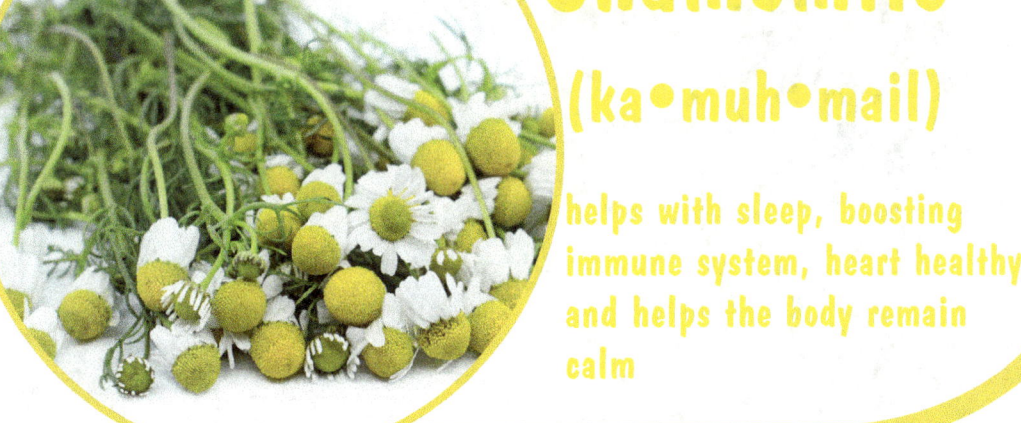

Chamomile
(ka•muh•mail)

helps with sleep, boosting immune system, heart healthy, and helps the body remain calm

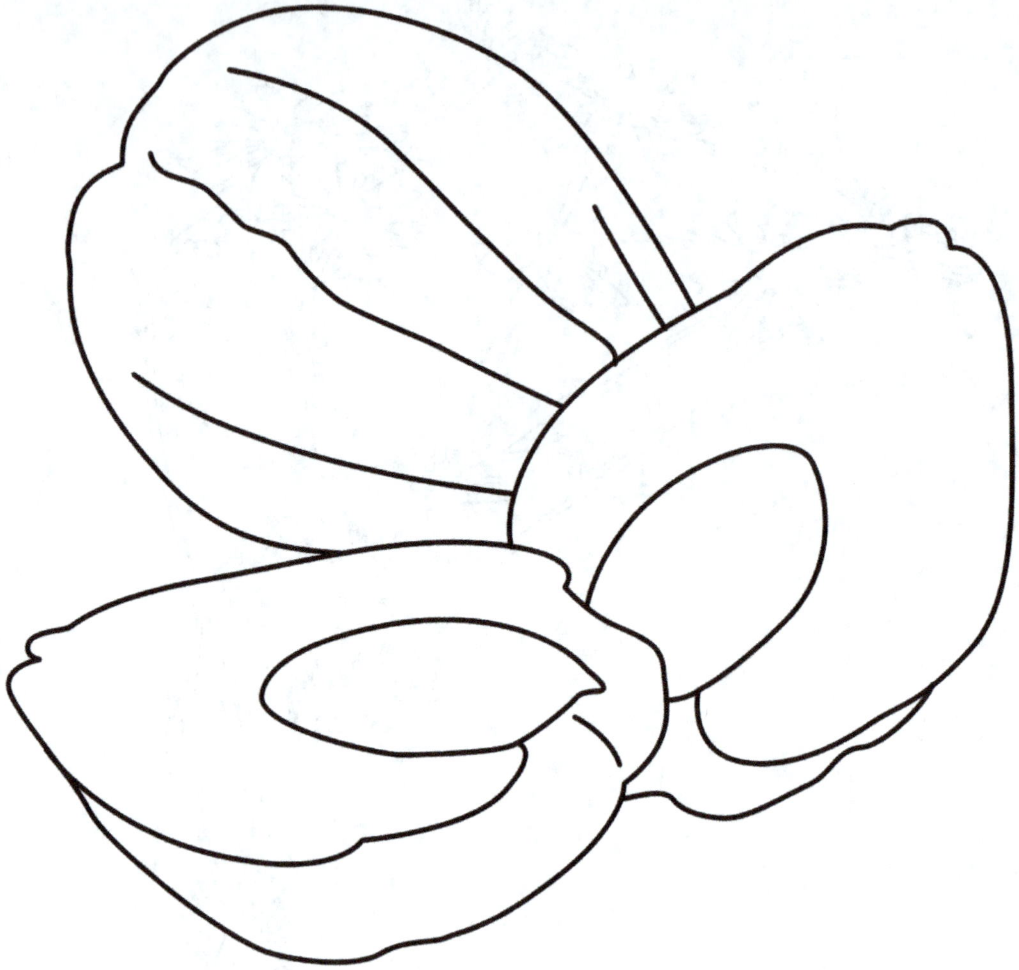

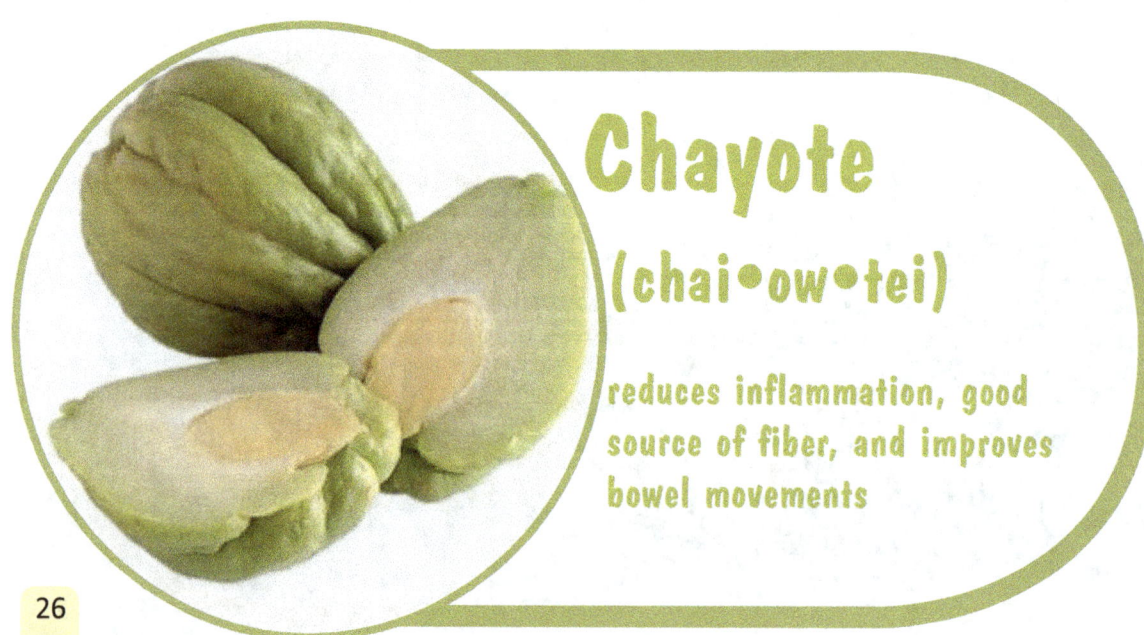

Chayote
(chai•ow•tei)

reduces inflammation, good source of fiber, and improves bowel movements

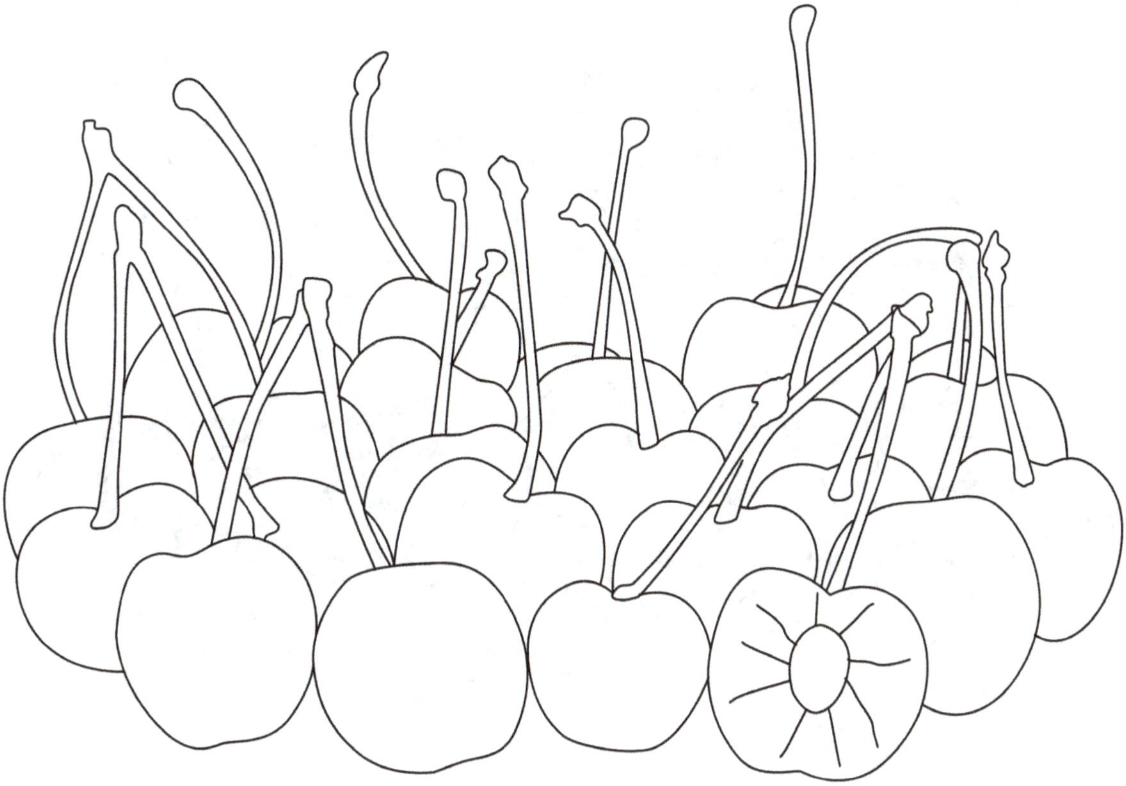

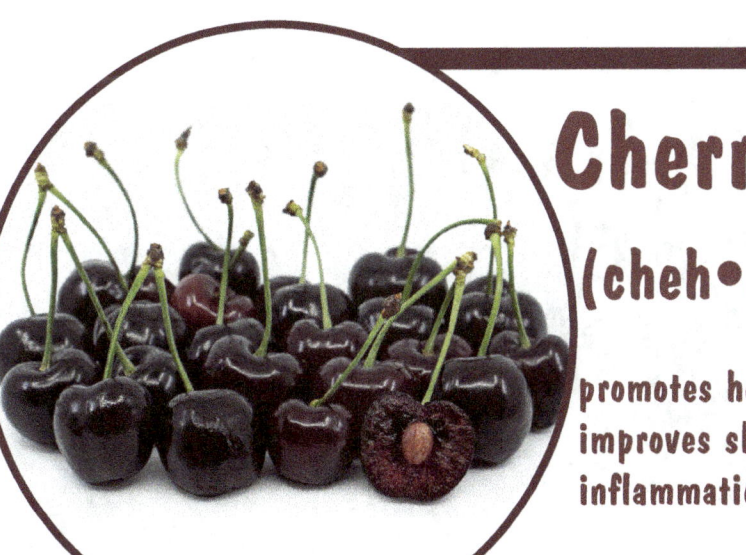

Cherries
(cheh•reez)

promotes heart and brain health, improves sleep, reduces inflammation and chronic pain

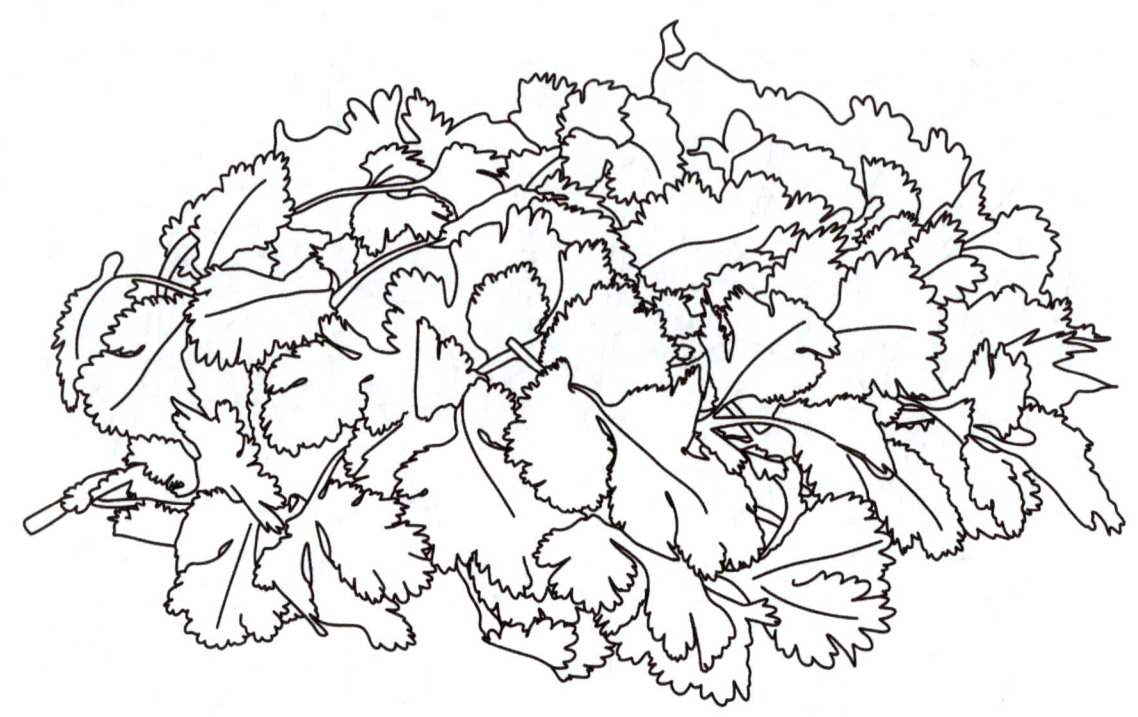

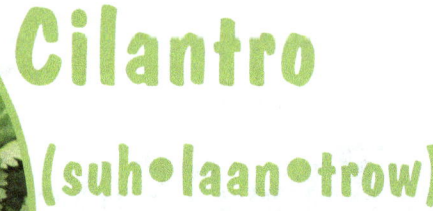

Cilantro
(suh•laan•trow)

rids the body of heavy metals, improves sleep, anti-inflammatory, helps reduce muscle spasms

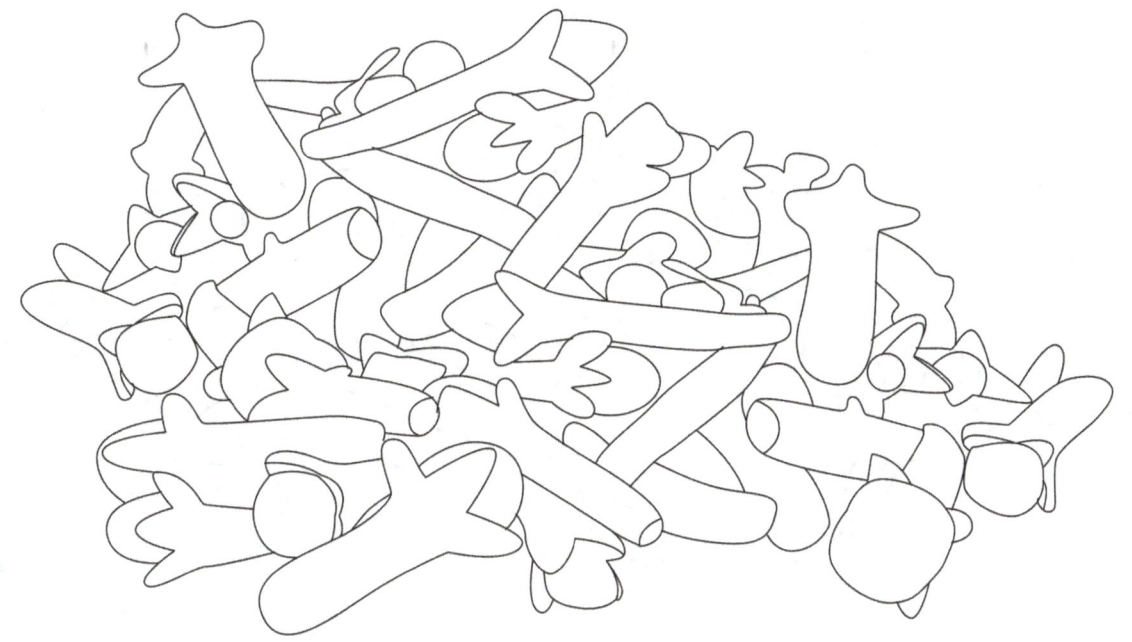

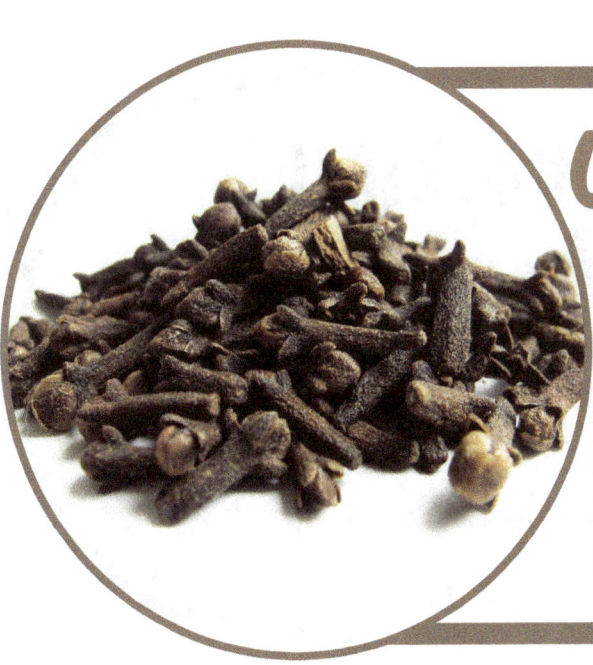

Cloves
(klowvz)

high in antioxidants, helps the liver and bones, prevents stomach pain, and helps kill bacteria

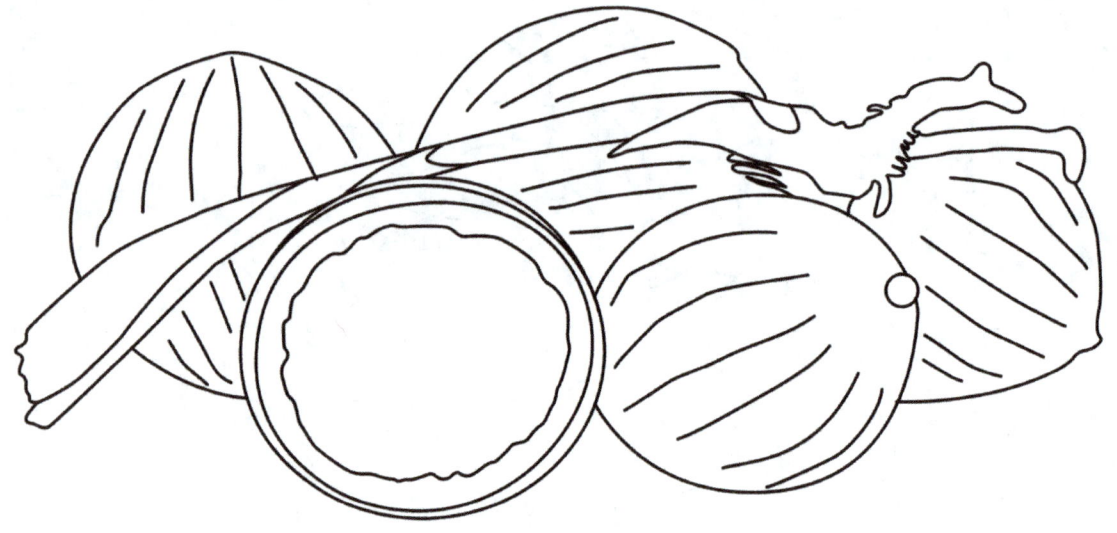

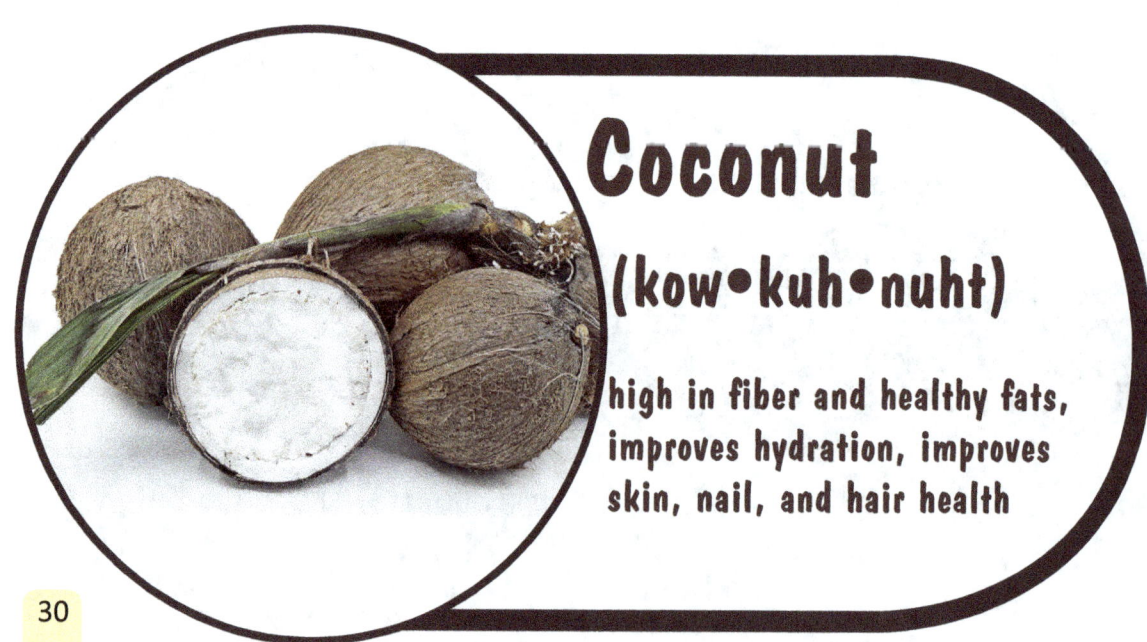

Coconut
(kow•kuh•nuht)

high in fiber and healthy fats, improves hydration, improves skin, nail, and hair health

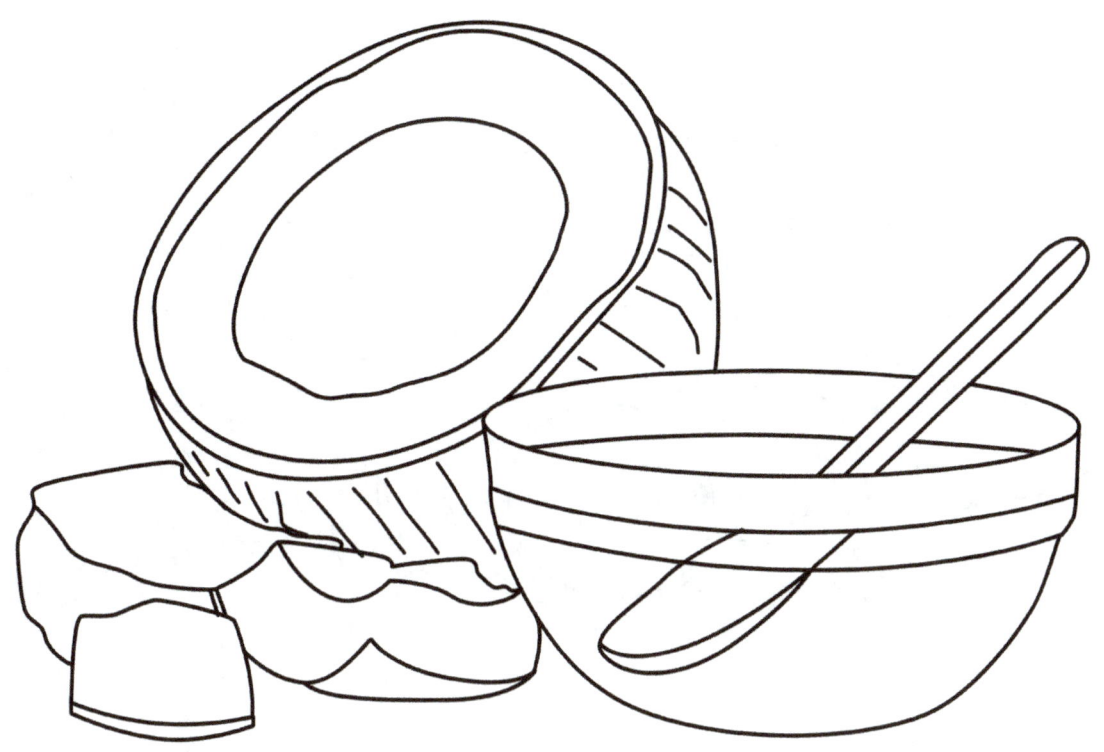

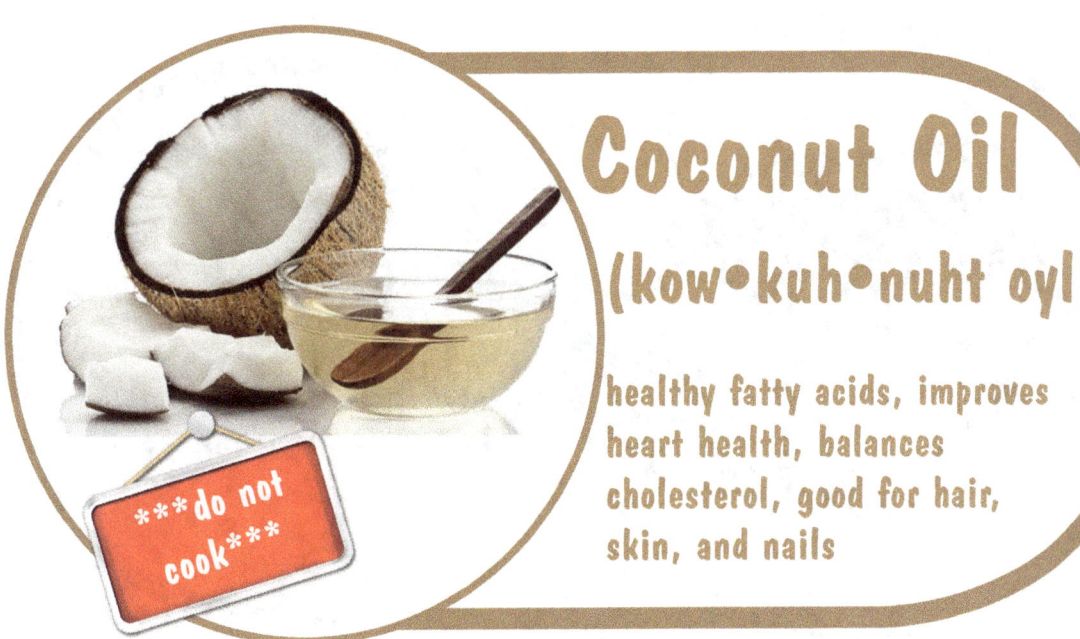

Coconut Oil
(kow•kuh•nuht oyl)

healthy fatty acids, improves heart health, balances cholesterol, good for hair, skin, and nails

do not cook

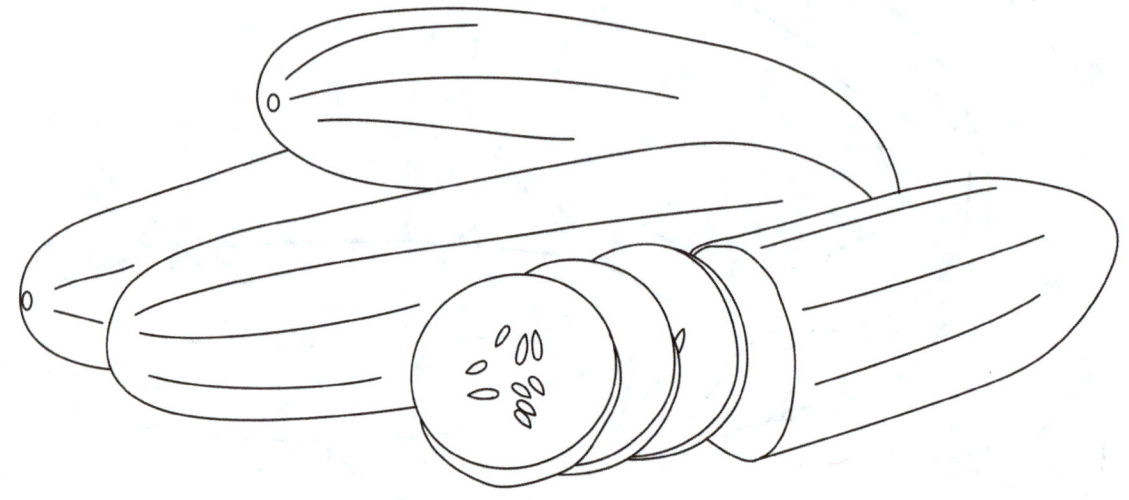

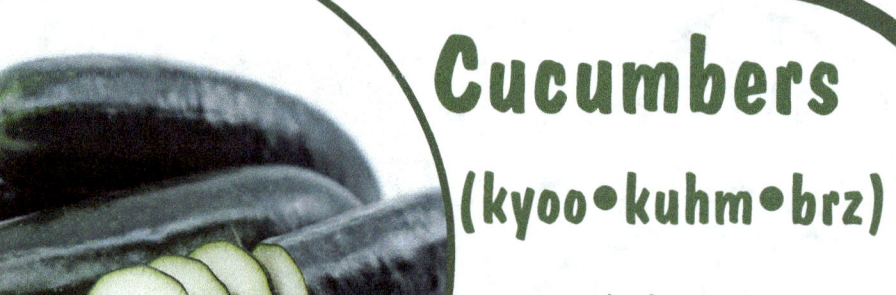

Cucumbers
(kyoo•kuhm•brz)

promotes hydration, regulates blood sugar, helpful for the skin and blood

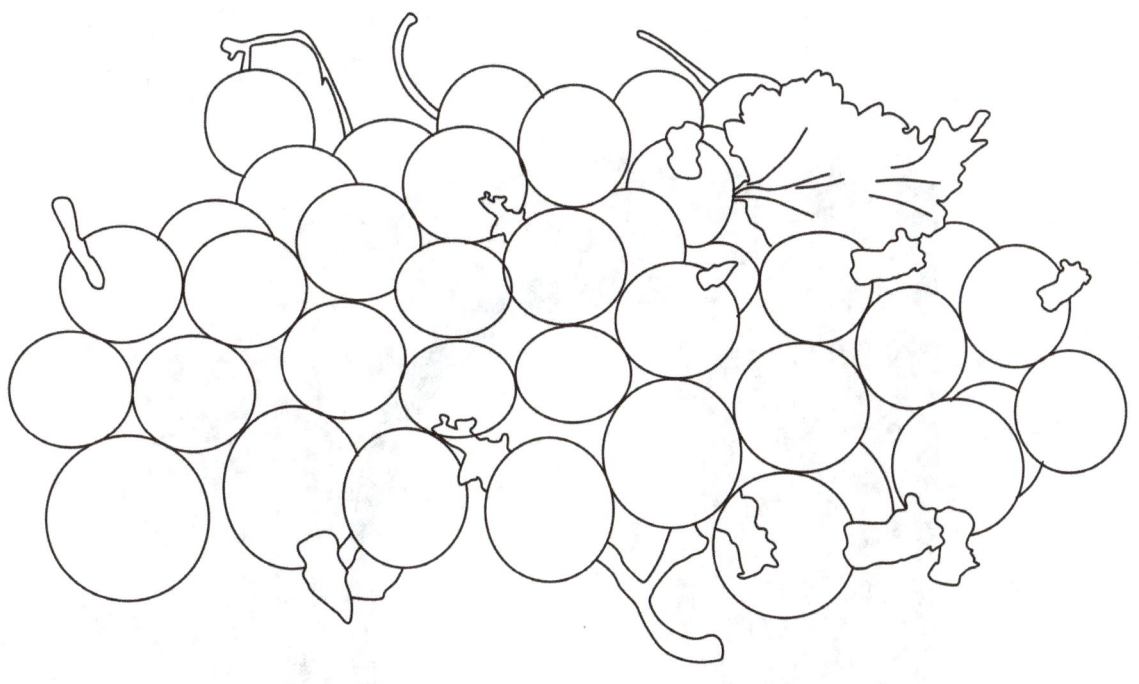

Currants
(kur•uhnts)

immune system booster, soothes coughs and sore throat, reduces symptoms of the flu, and good source of iron

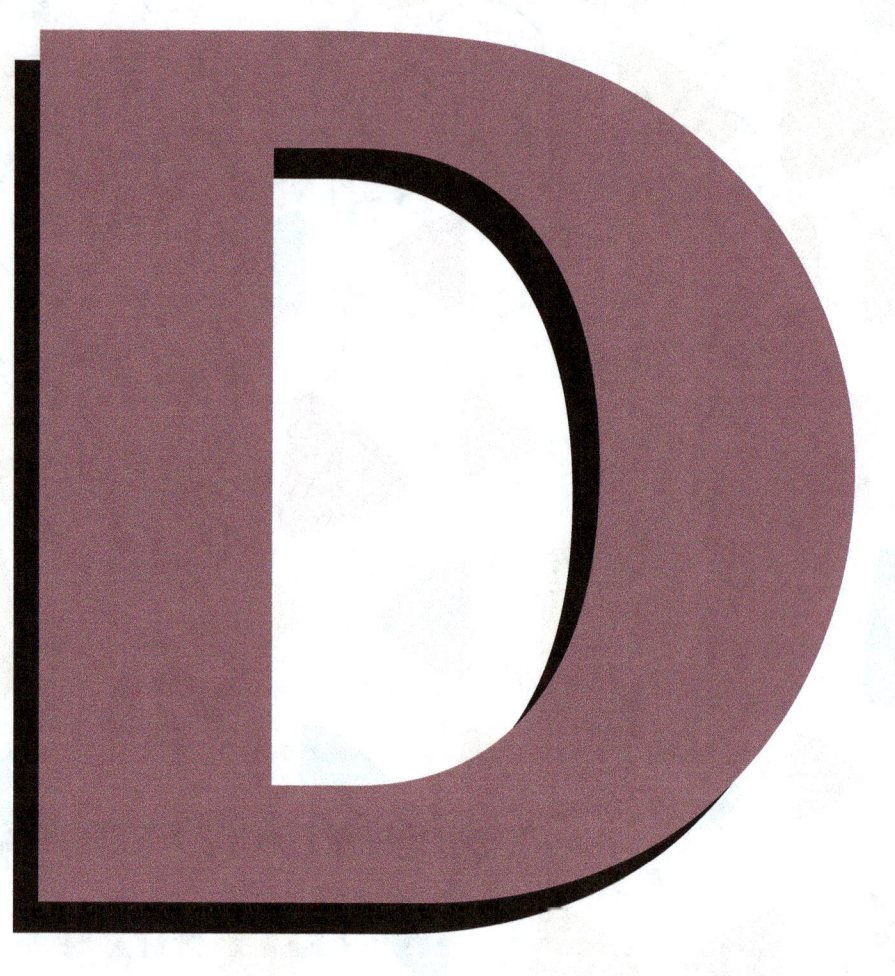

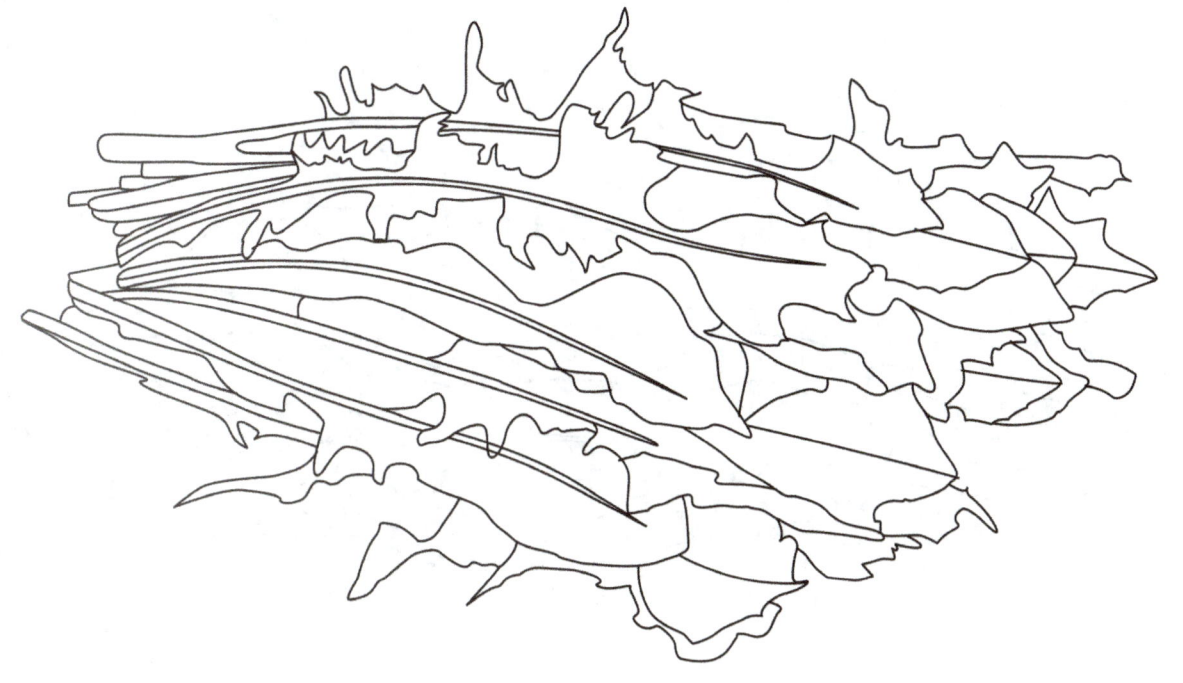

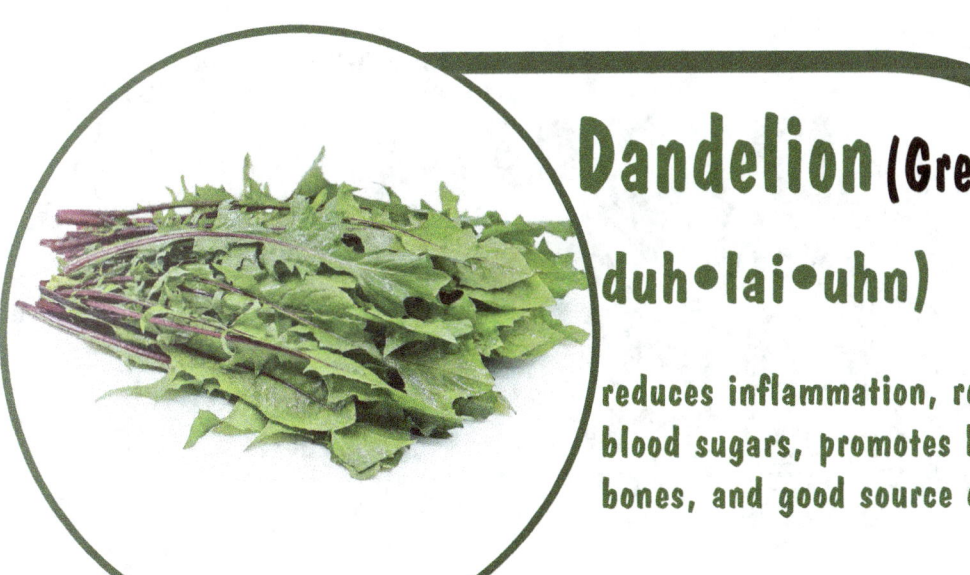

Dandelion (Greens)

(duh•lai•uhn)

reduces inflammation, regulates blood sugars, promotes healthy bones, and good source of iron

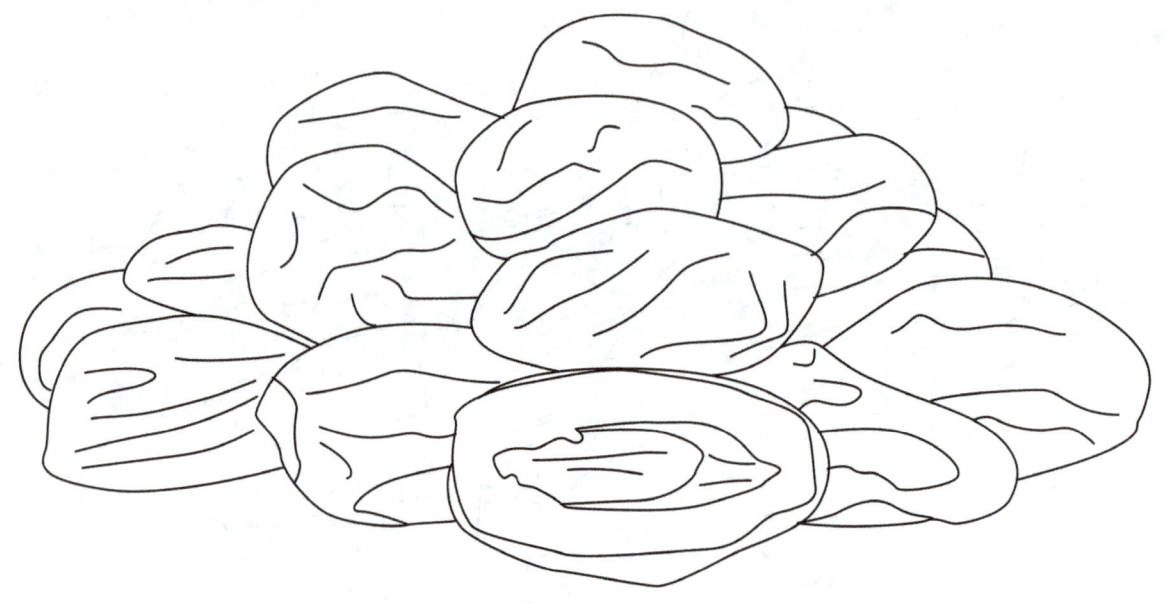

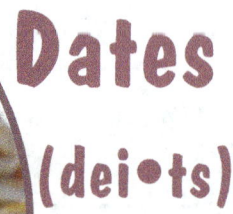

Dates
(dei•ts)

high in fiber, promotes brain health, and supports a healthy digestive tract

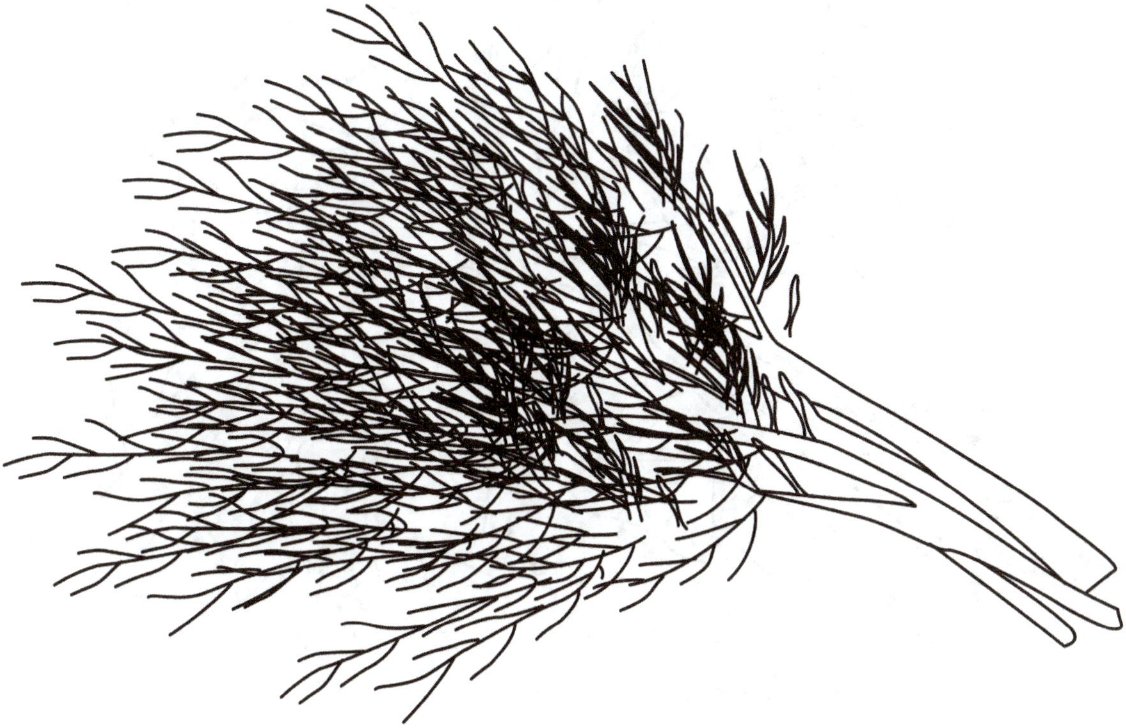

Dill
(dil)

source of fiber, helps build strong bones, good for skin, and helps prevent heart diseases

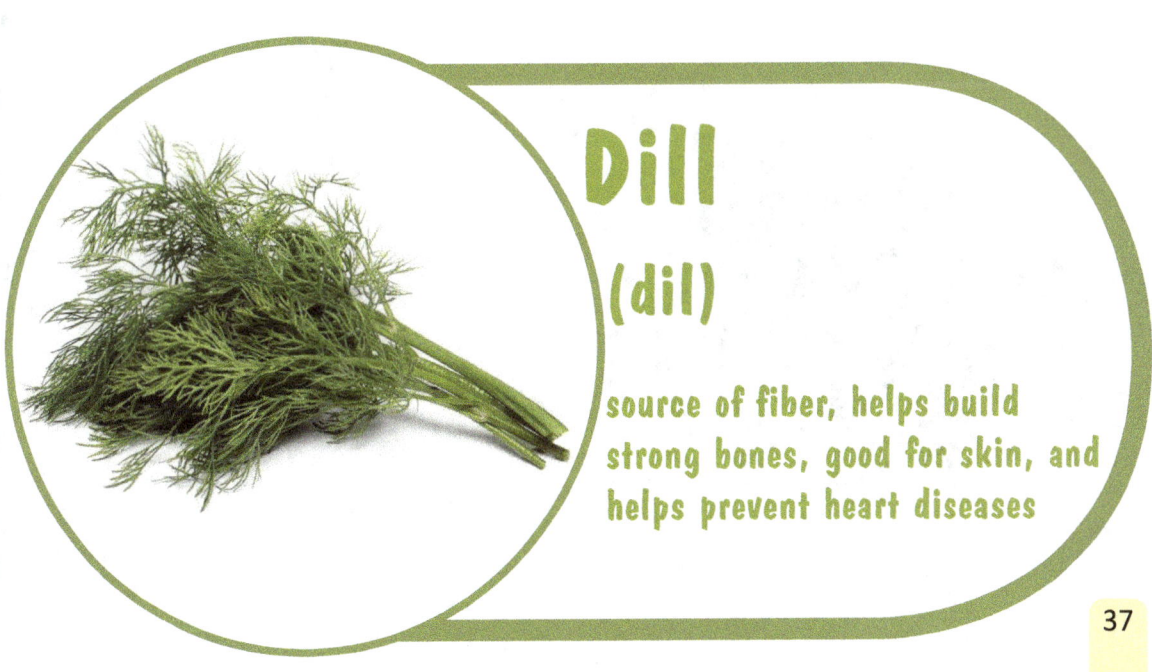

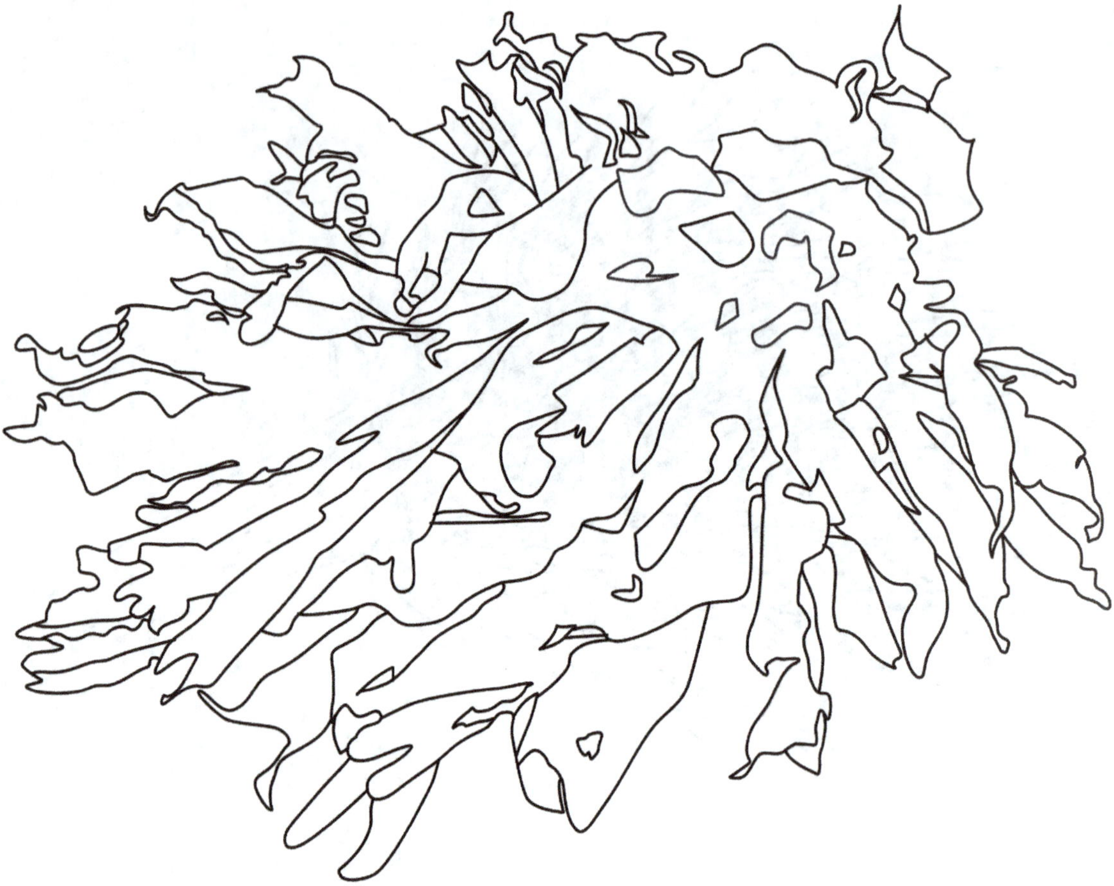

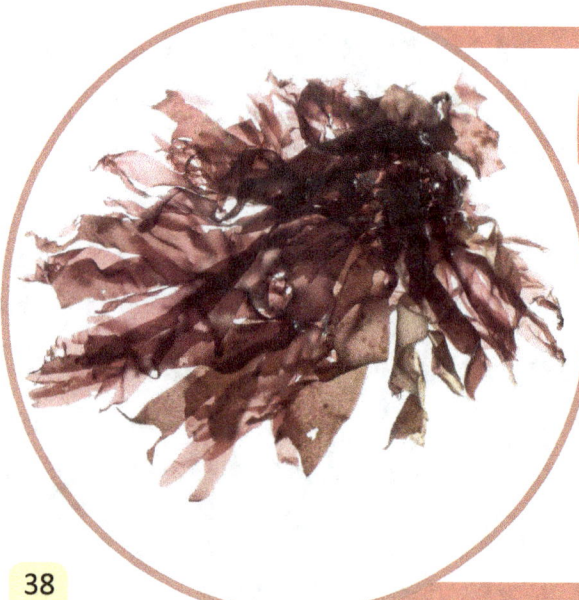

Dulse
(duhls•e)

strengthens bones, improves eyesight, lowers blood pressure, and good source of healthy fats.

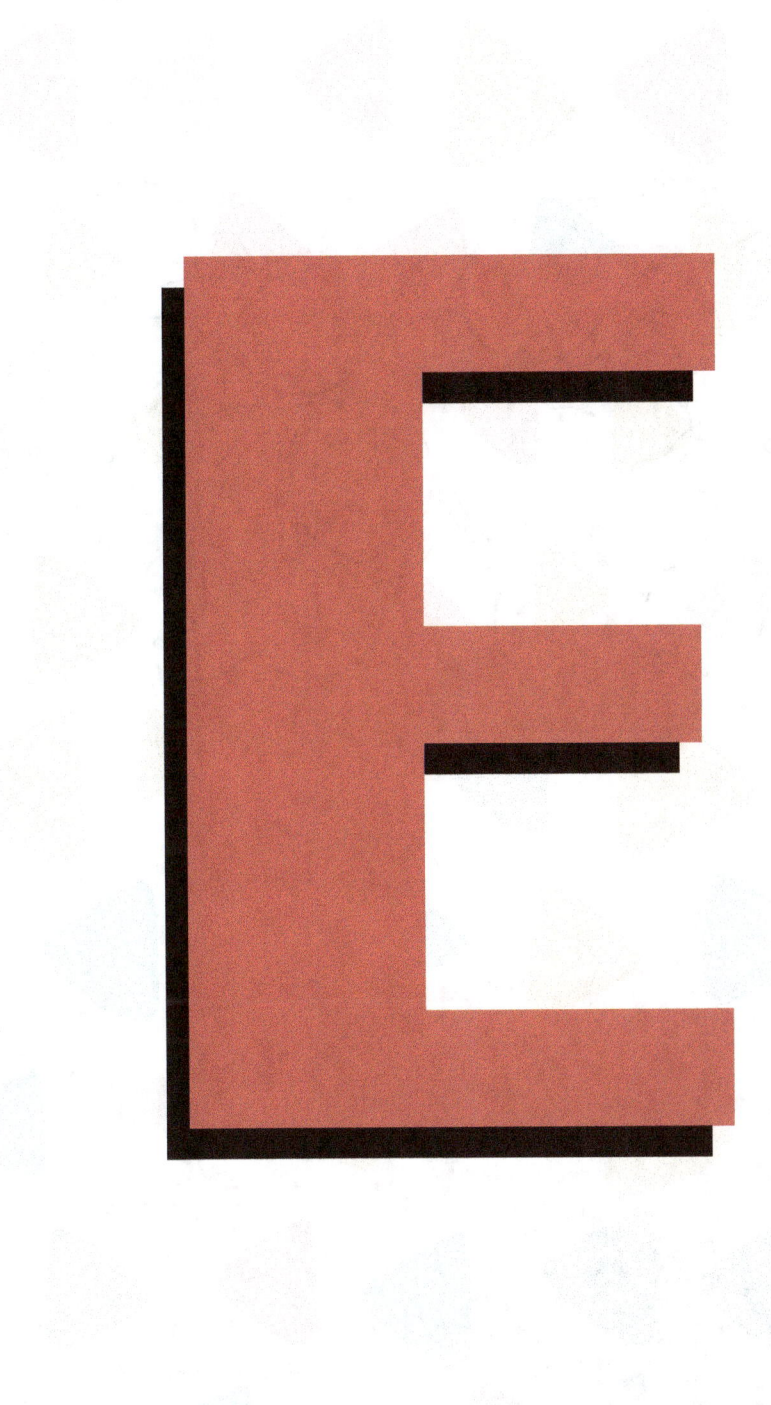

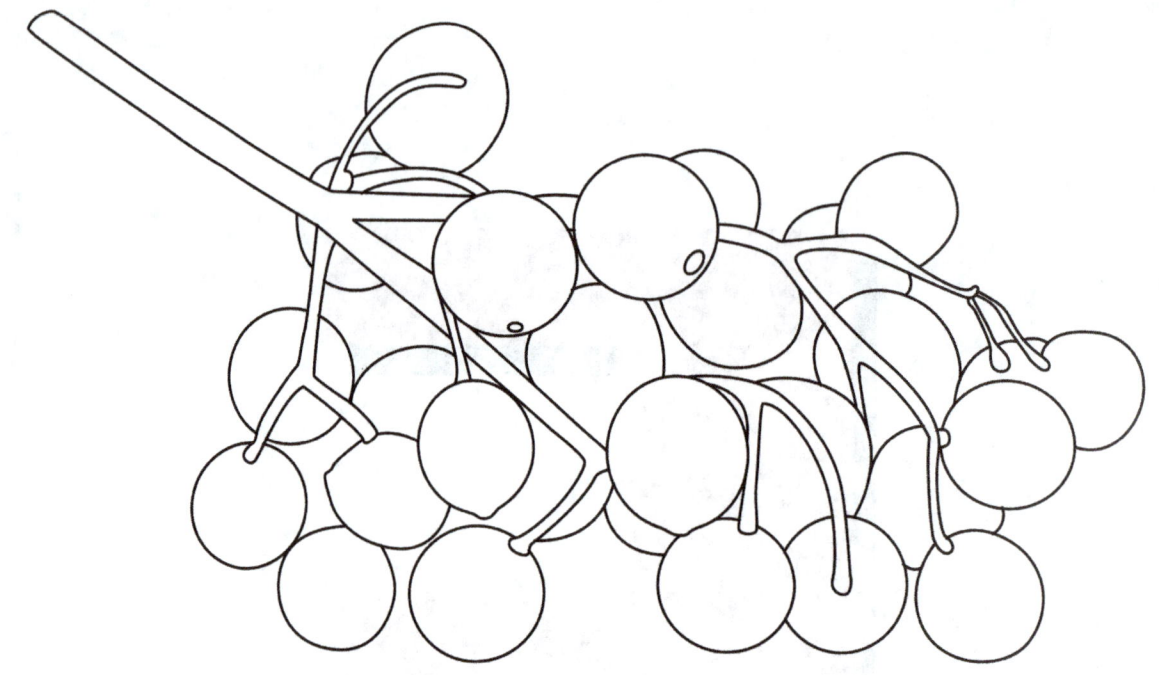

Elderberry
(el•dr•beh•ree)

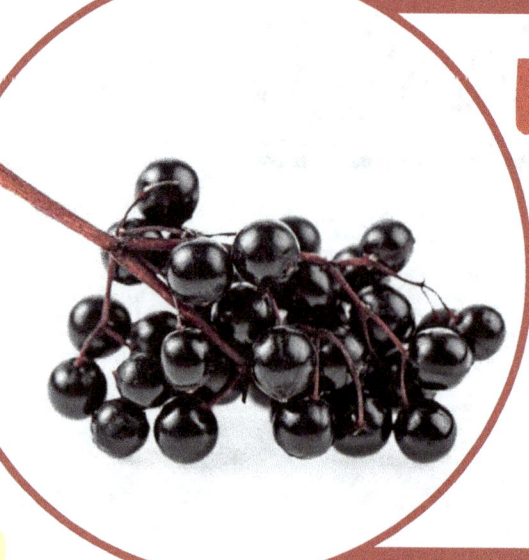

boosts immune system, reduce inflammation, and relieves colds, coughs, and symptoms of the flu

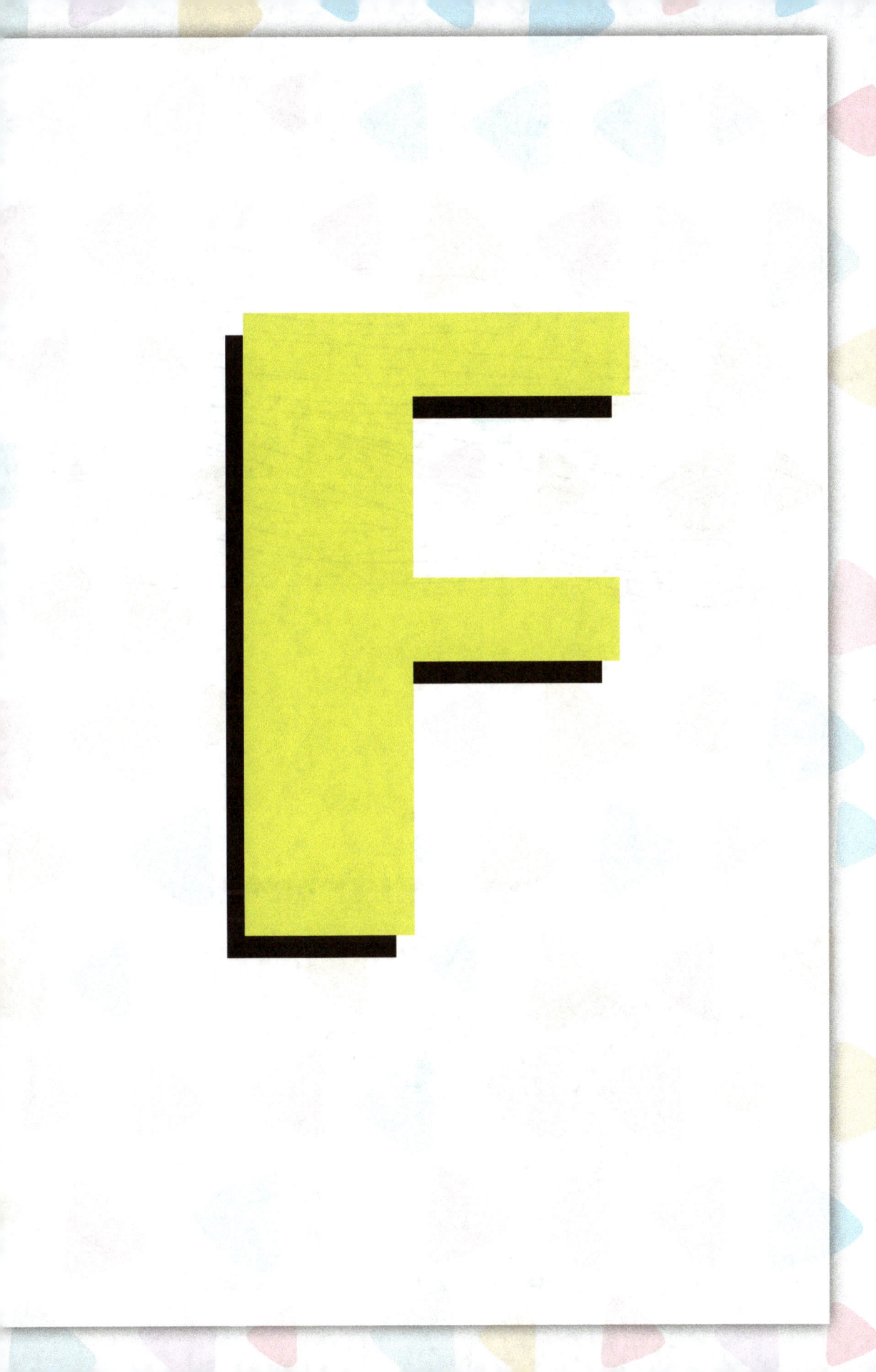

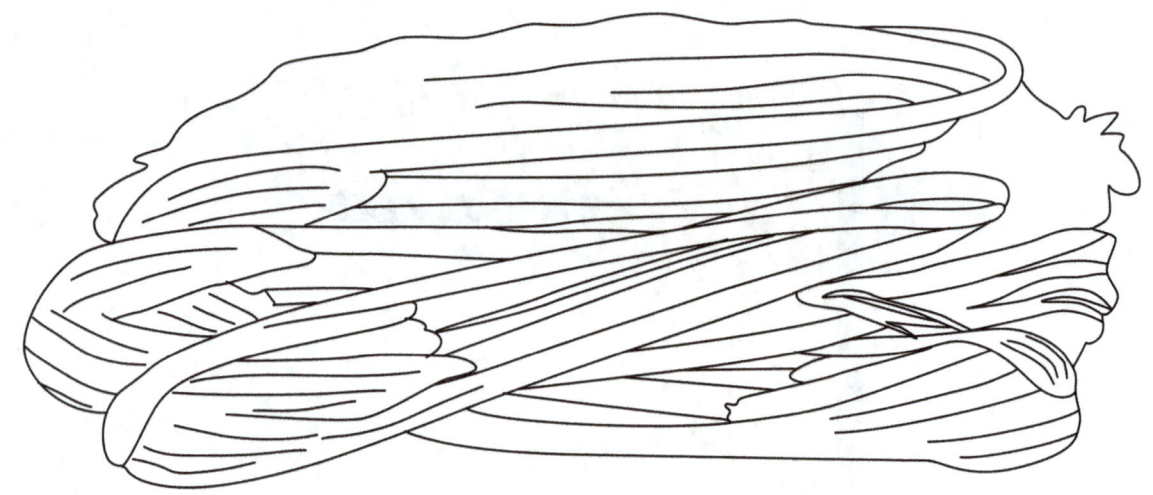

Fennel
(feh•nuhl)

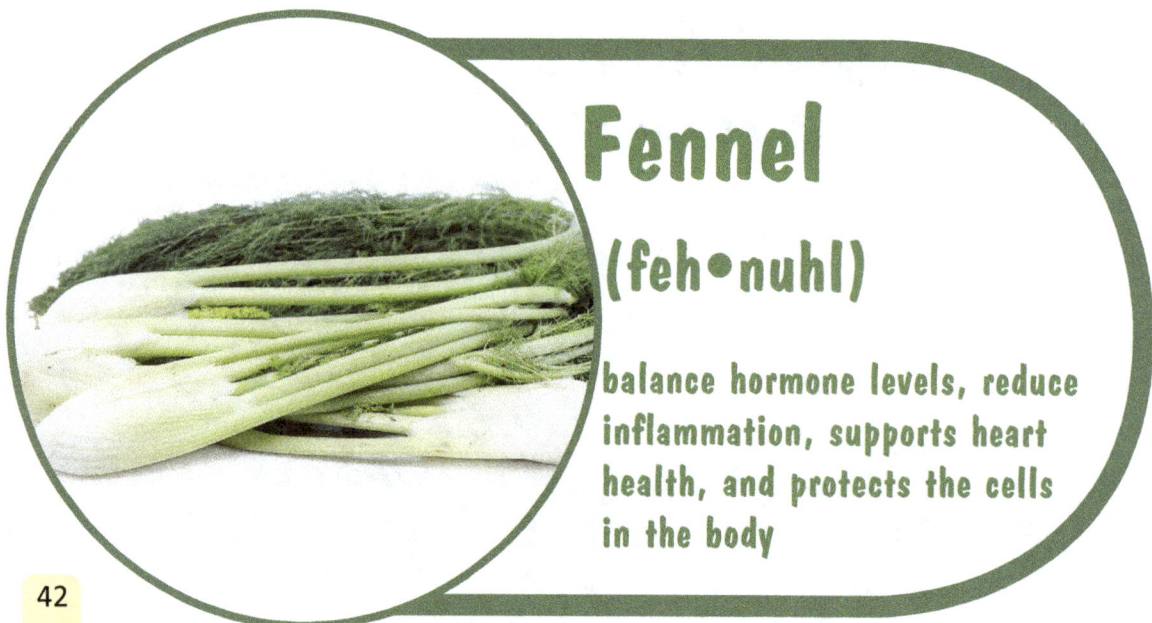

balance hormone levels, reduce inflammation, supports heart health, and protects the cells in the body

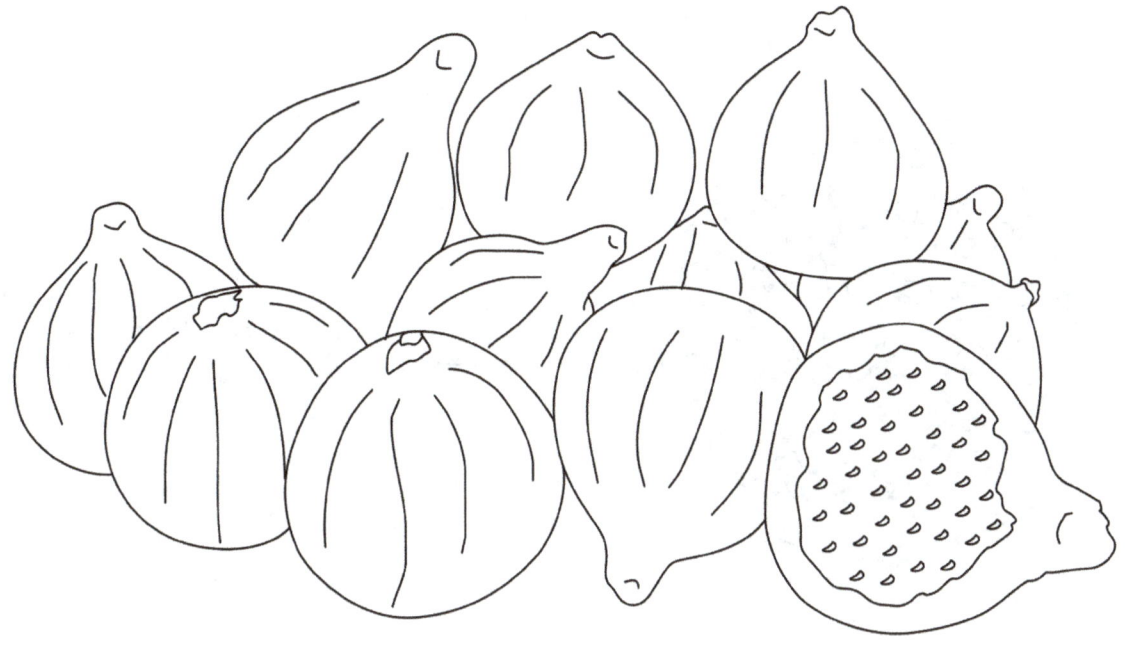

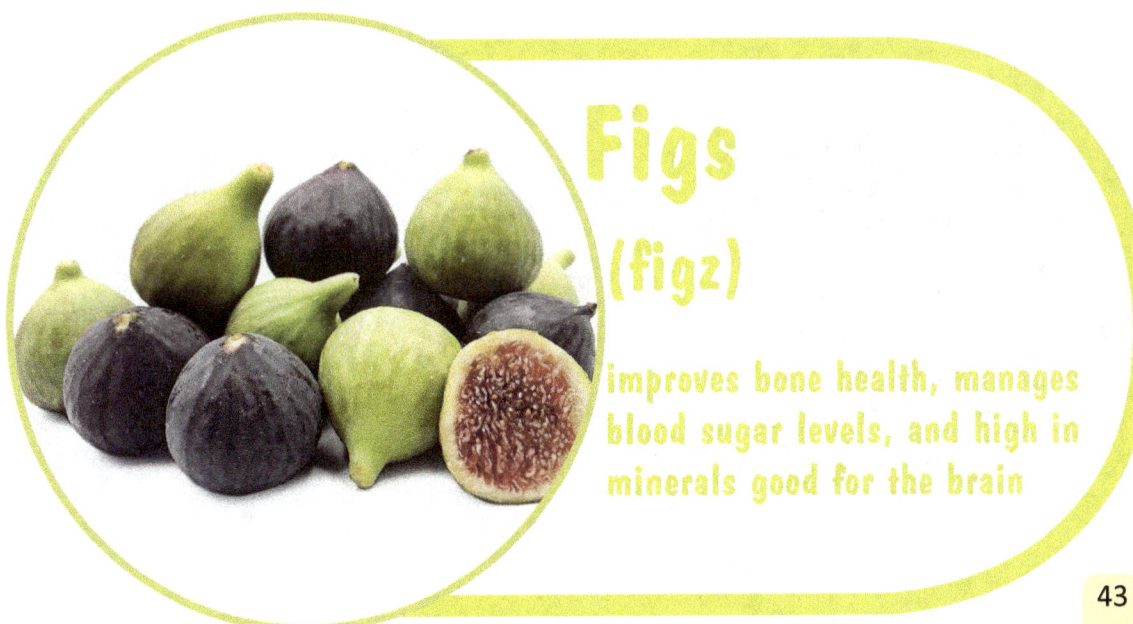

Figs
(figz)

improves bone health, manages blood sugar levels, and high in minerals good for the brain

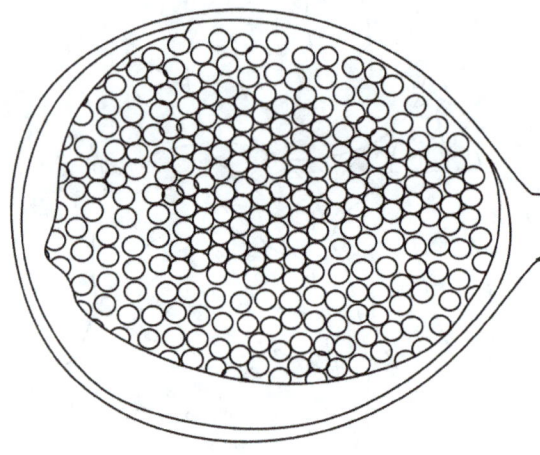

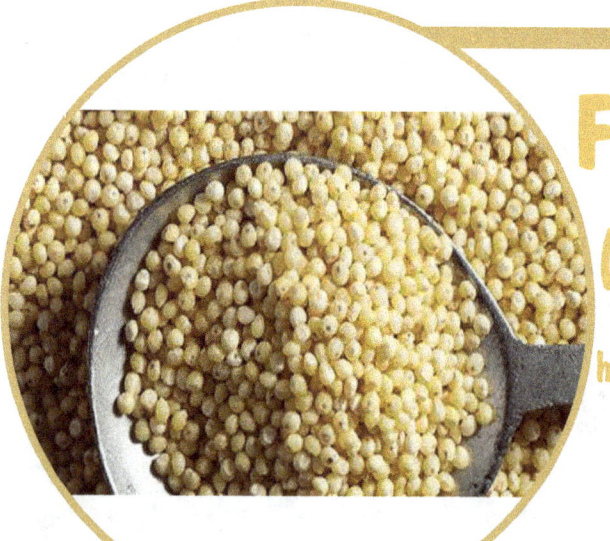

Fonio
(fo•nee•o)

helps digestion, improve energy

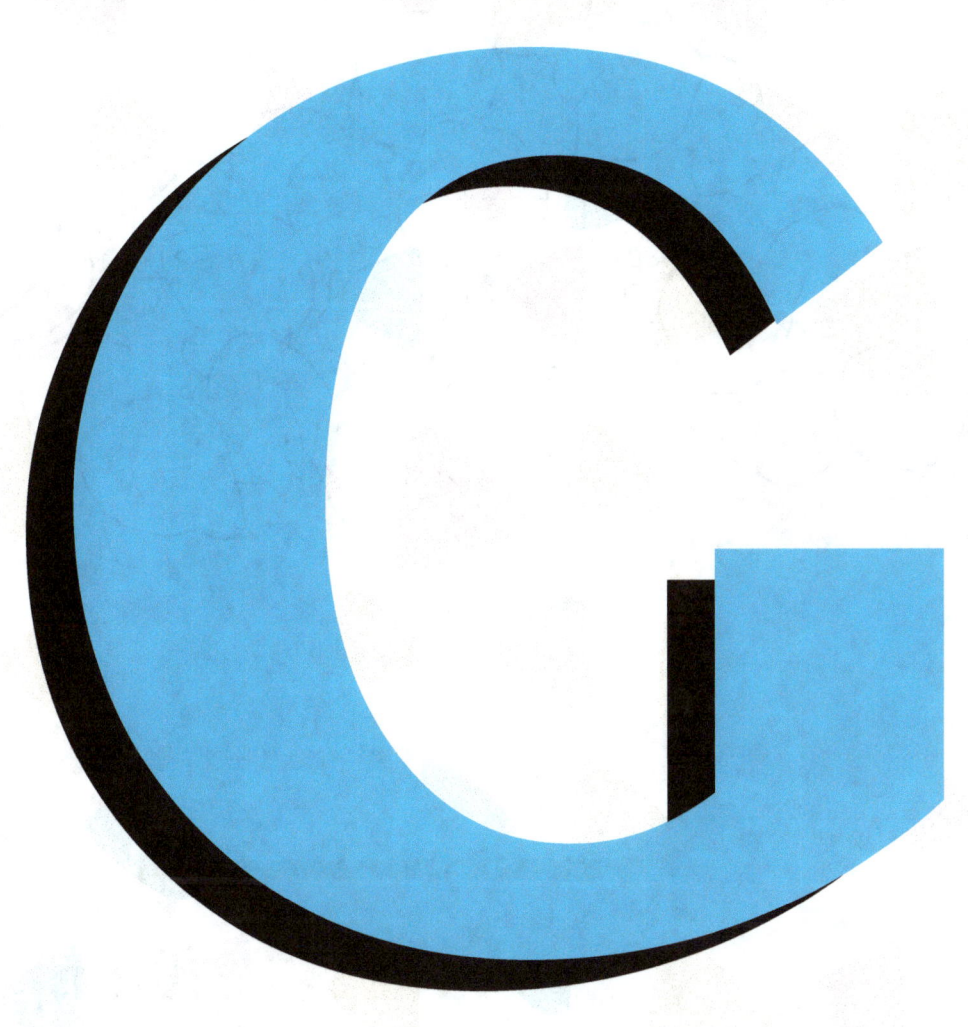

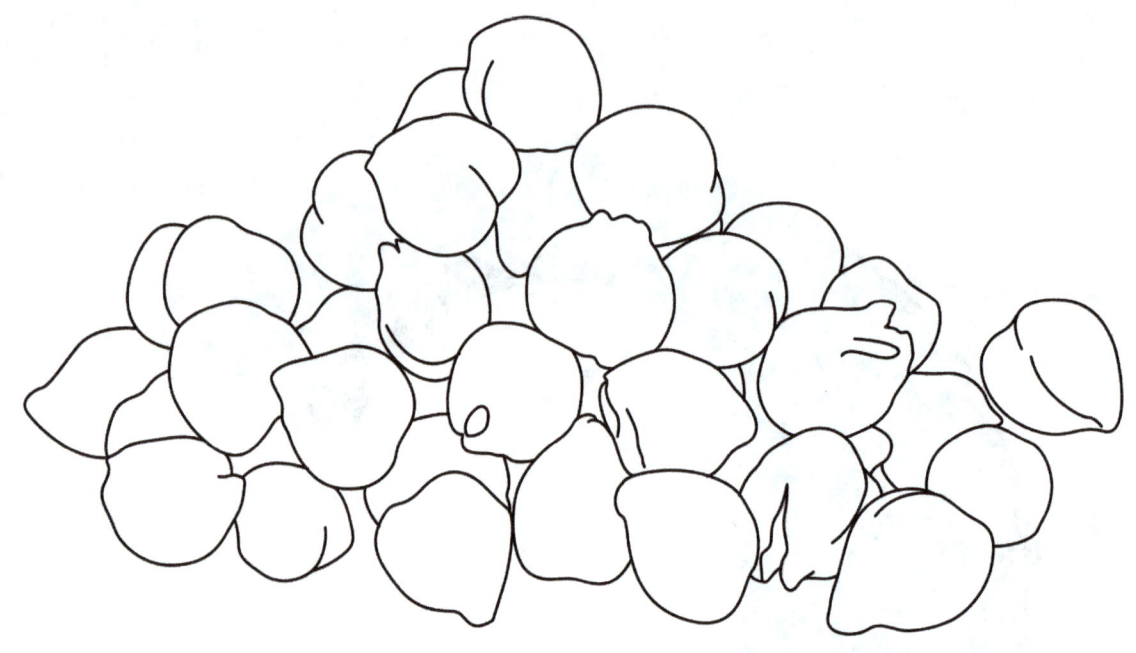

Garbanzo (Beans)

(gaar•baan•zow)

high in fiber and amino acids needed for muscle growth, boosts energy, and regulates blood pressure levels

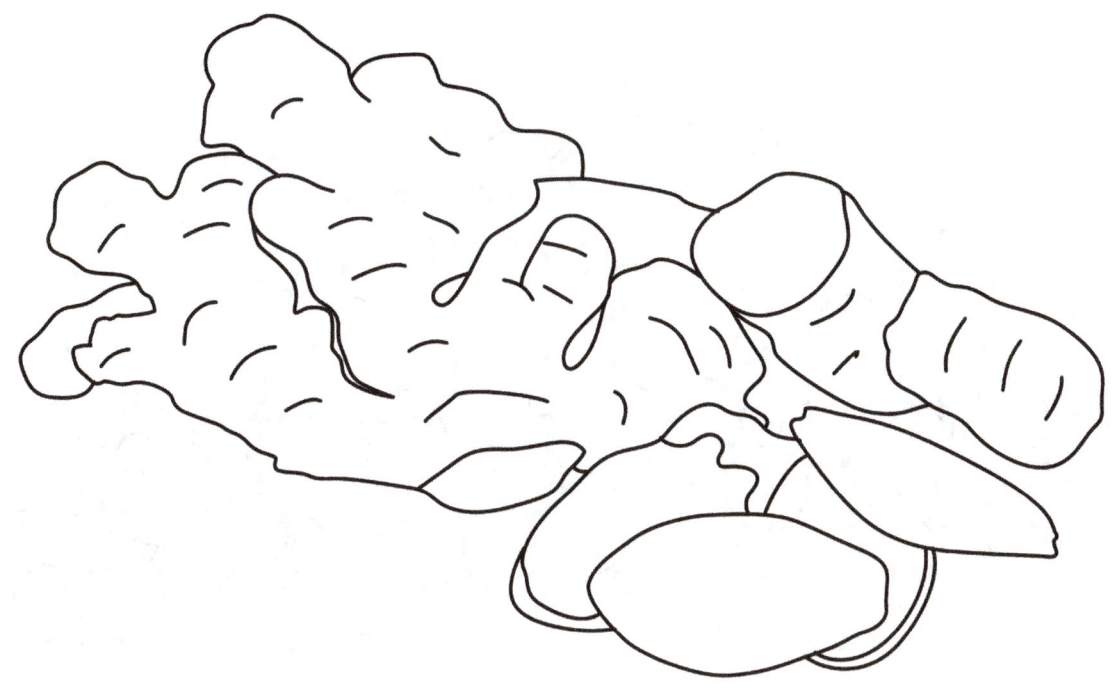

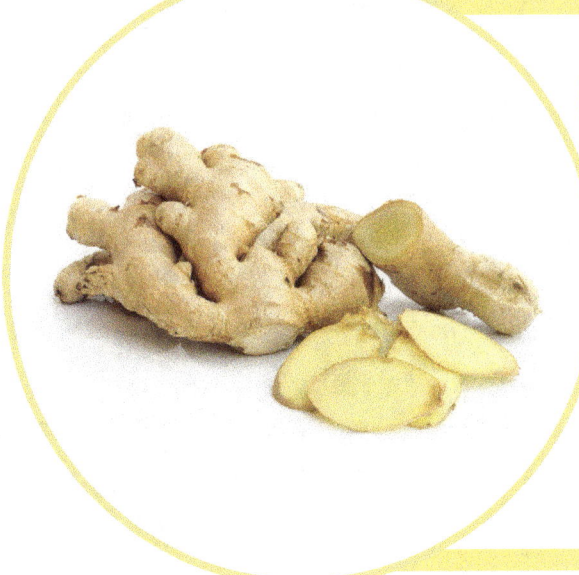

Ginger
(jin•jr)

immune system booster, reduces inflammation, and helps kill unhealthy bacteria that leads to sickness

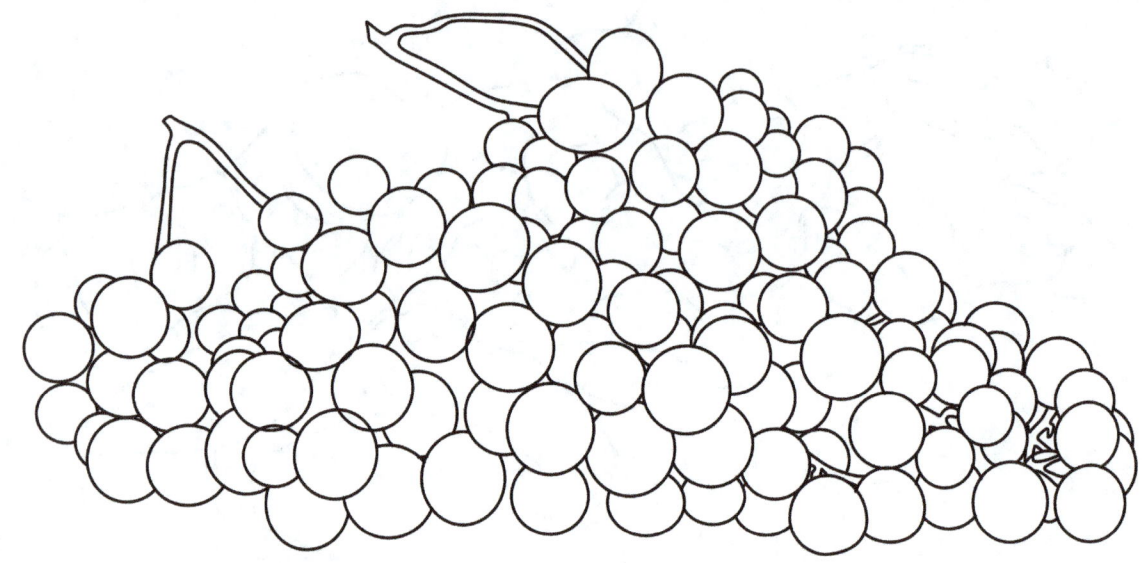

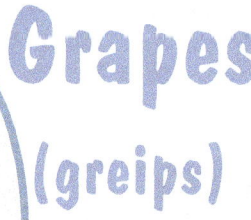

Grapes
(greips)

immune system booster, protects against harmful bacteria, and balances blood sugar levels

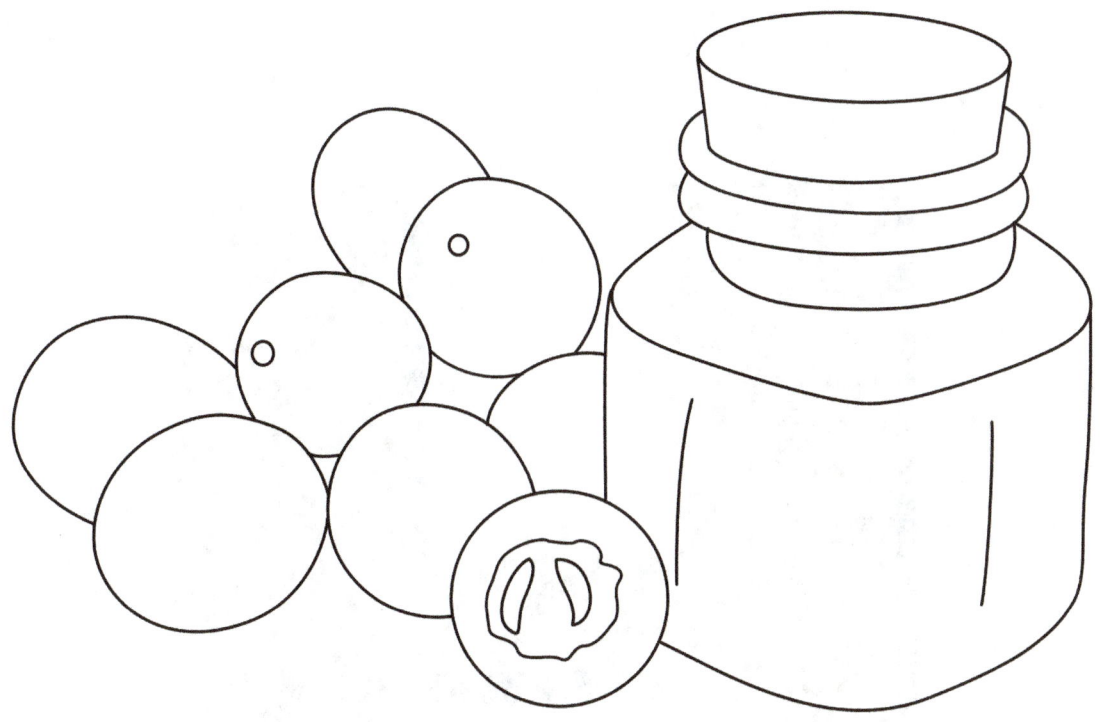

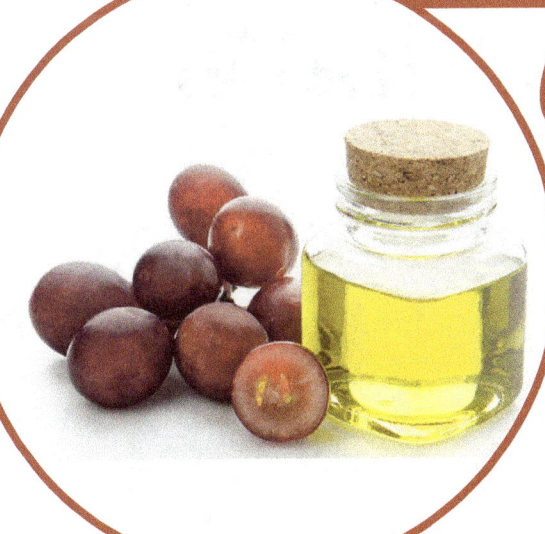

Grapeseed Oil
(greip•seed oyl)

repairs damaged cells and great for skin health

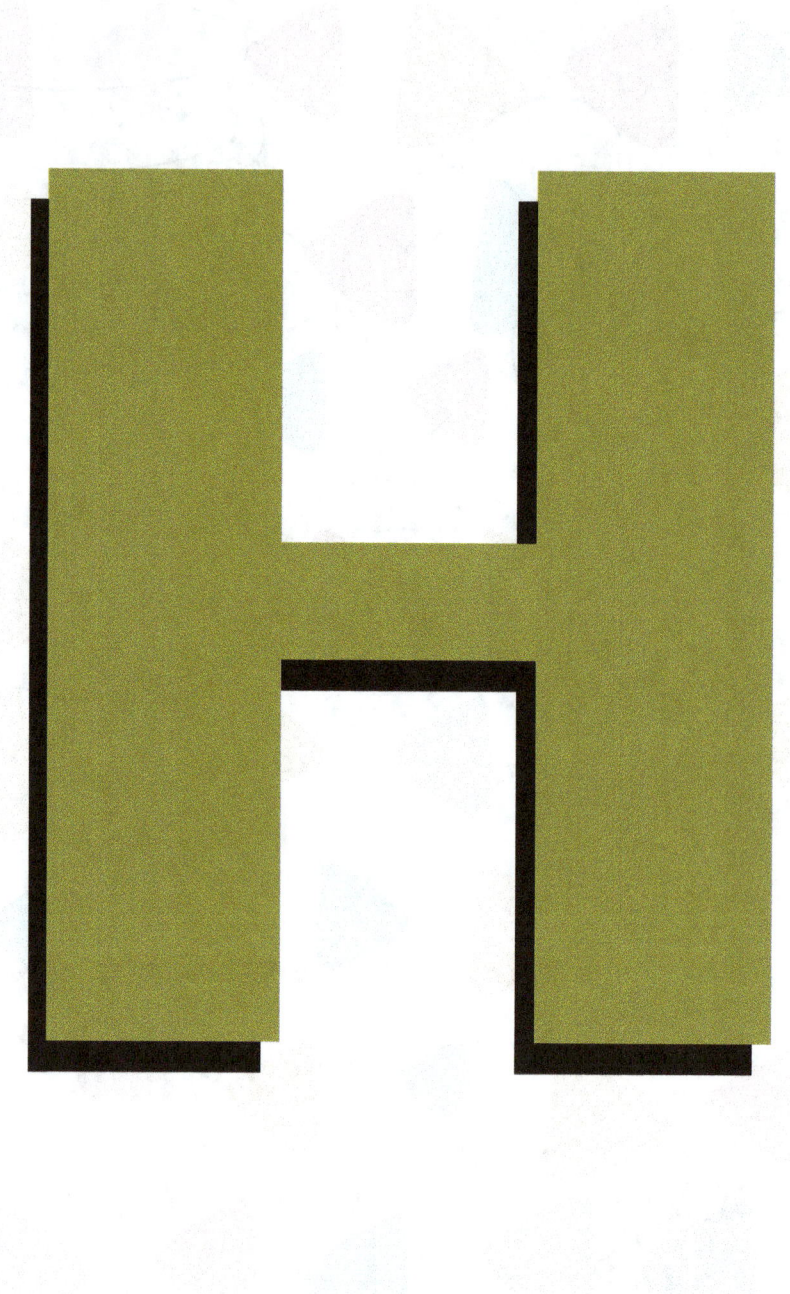

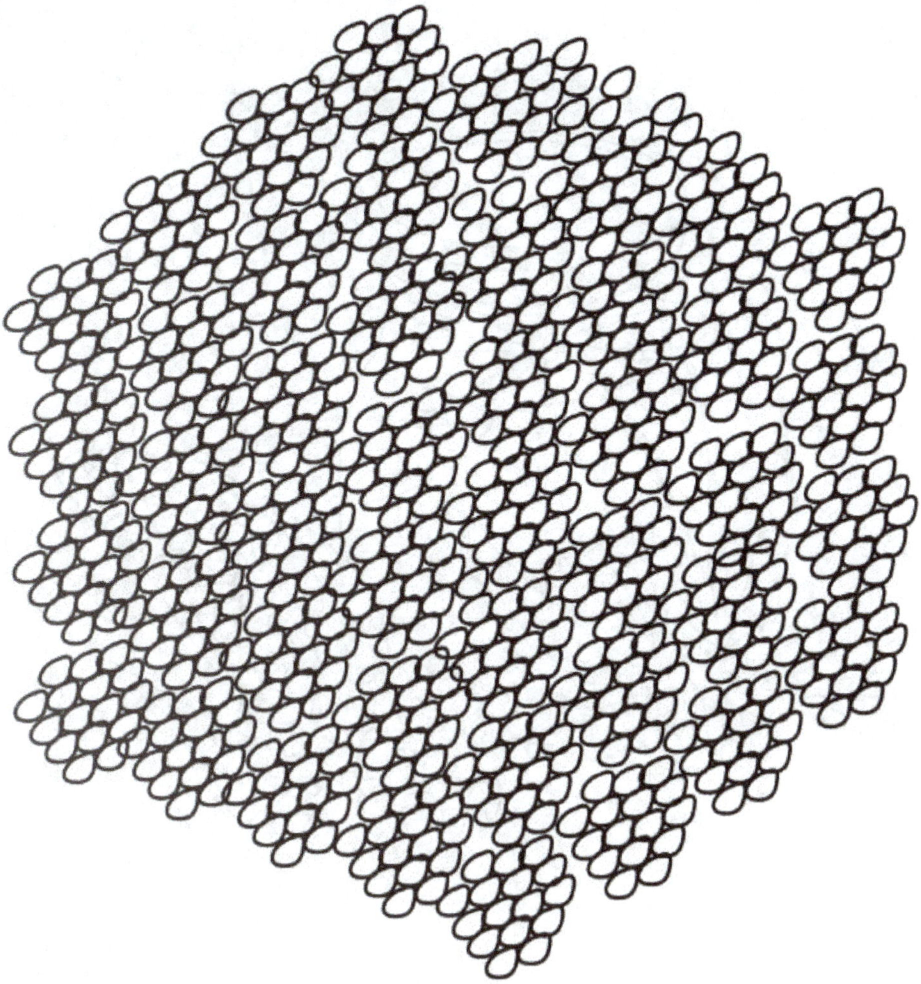

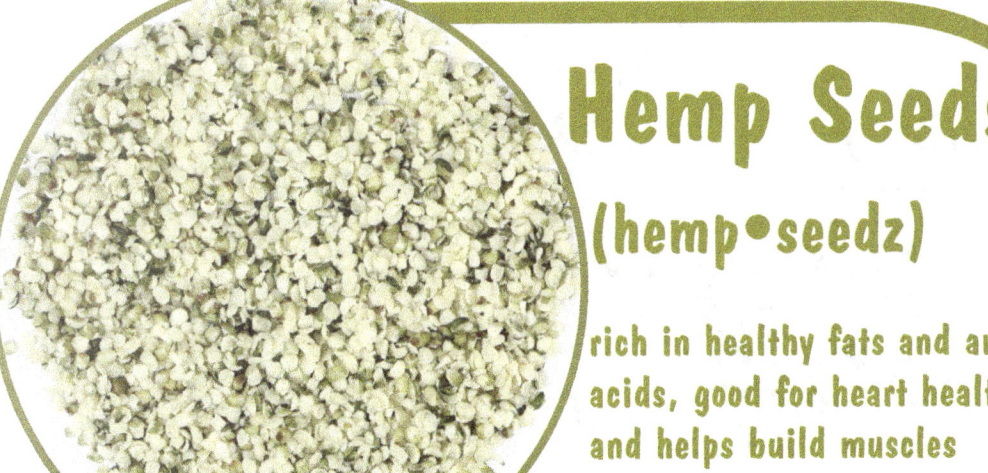

Hemp Seeds
(hemp•seedz)

rich in healthy fats and amino acids, good for heart health, and helps build muscles

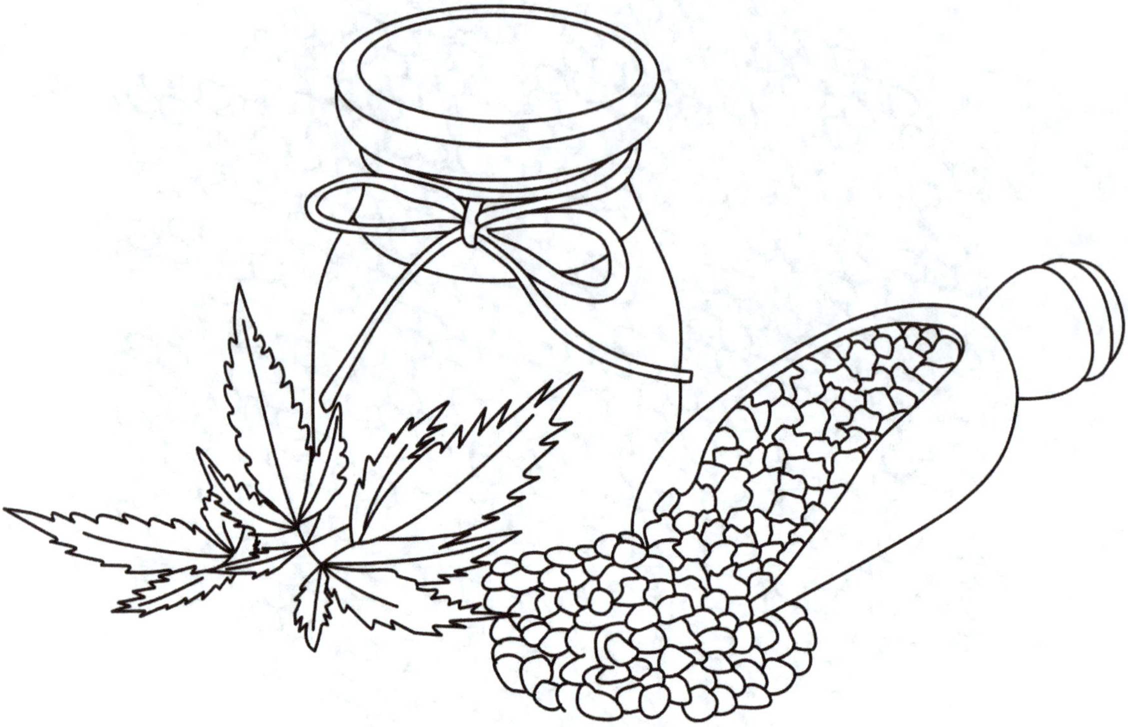

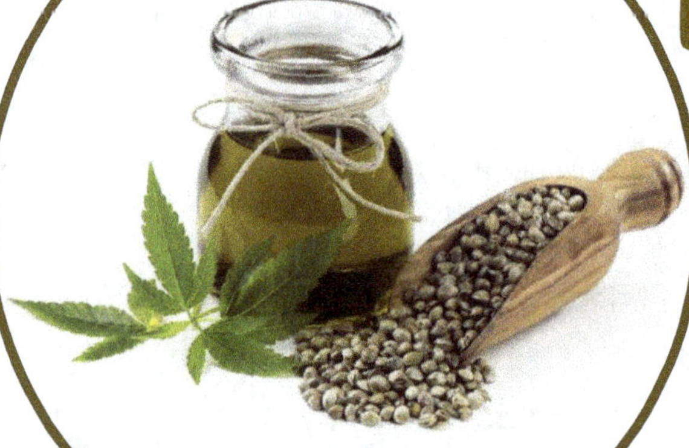

Hemp Seed Oil
(hemp seed oyl)

reduce risk for heart disease, improves sleep, and helps reduce nerve and joint pain

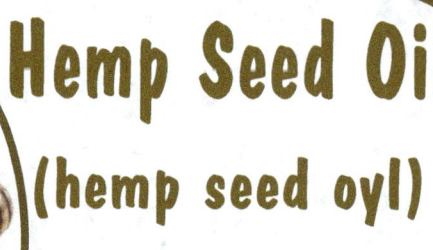

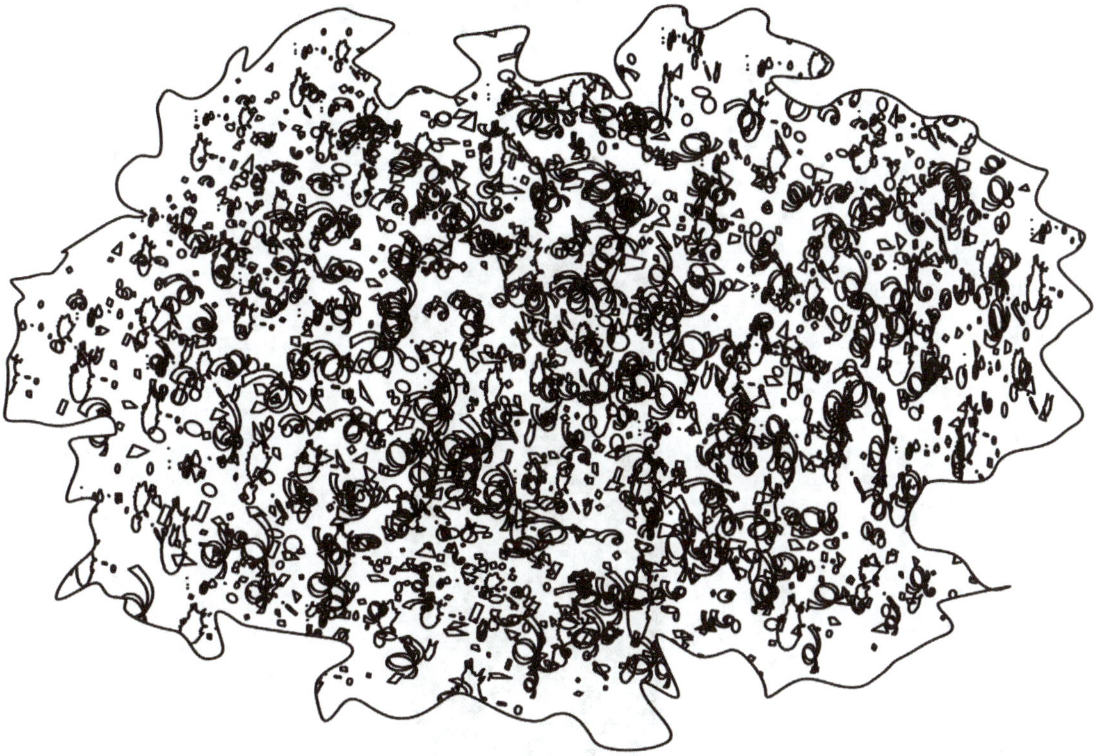

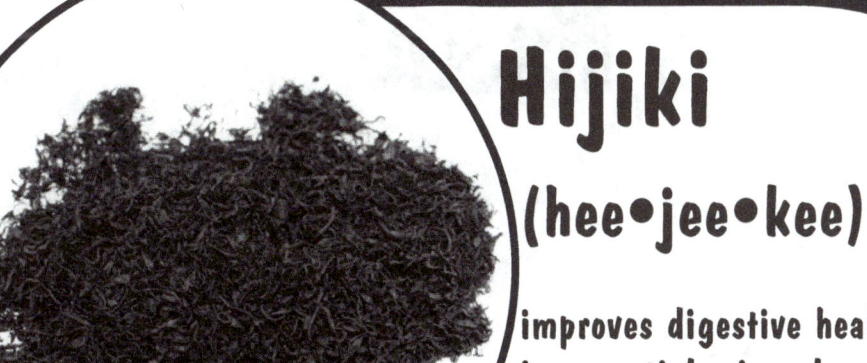

Hijiki
(hee•jee•kee)

improves digestive health, rich in essential minerals and dietary fiber

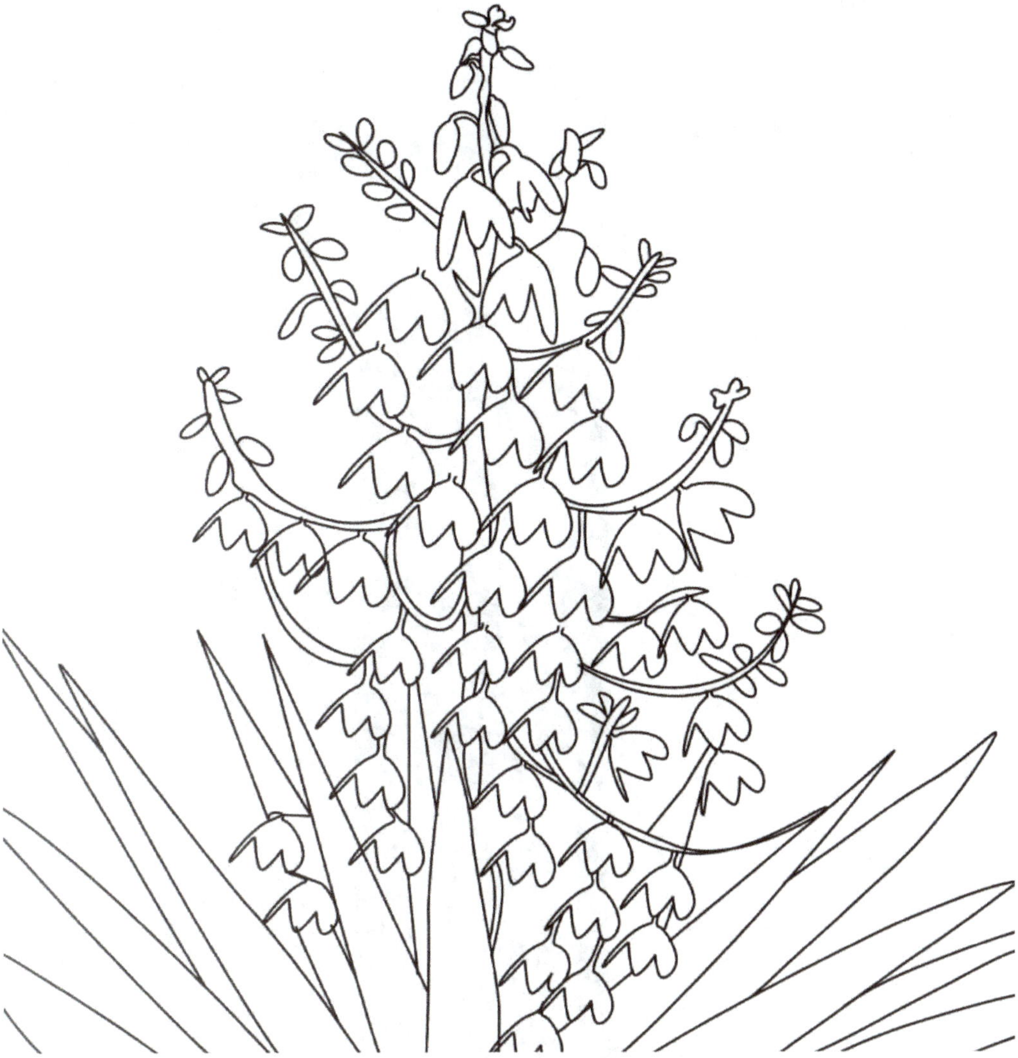

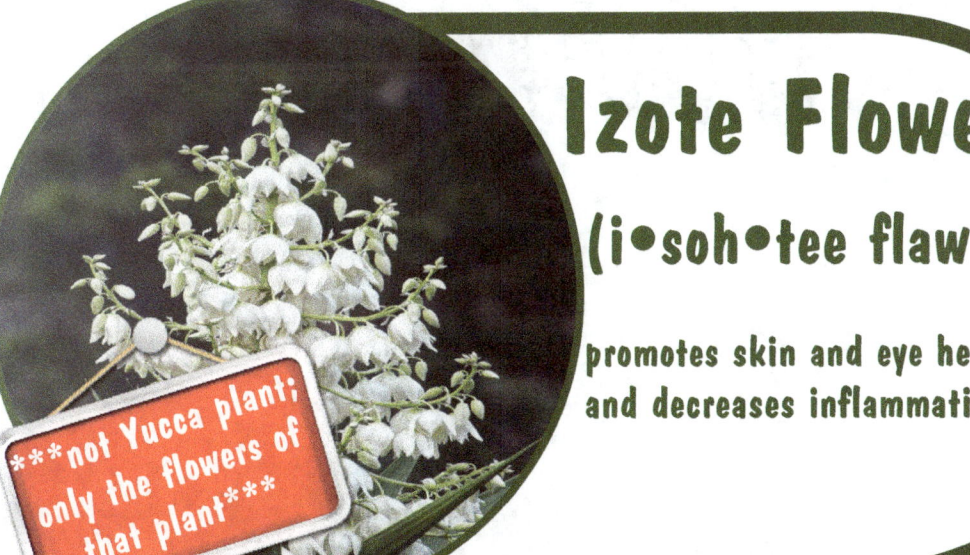

Izote Flower
(i•soh•tee flaw•ur)

promotes skin and eye health, and decreases inflammation

not Yucca plant; only the flowers of that plant

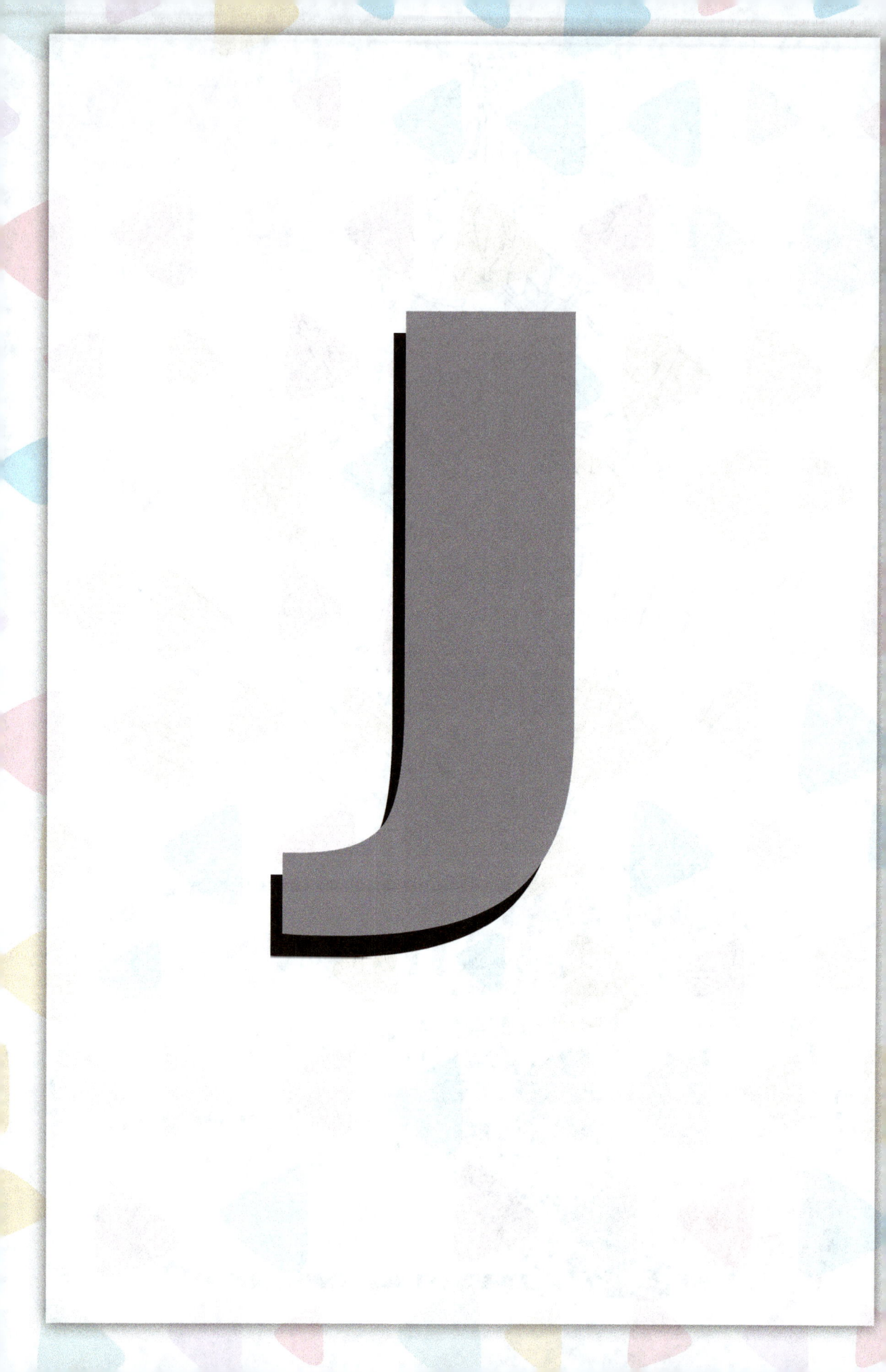

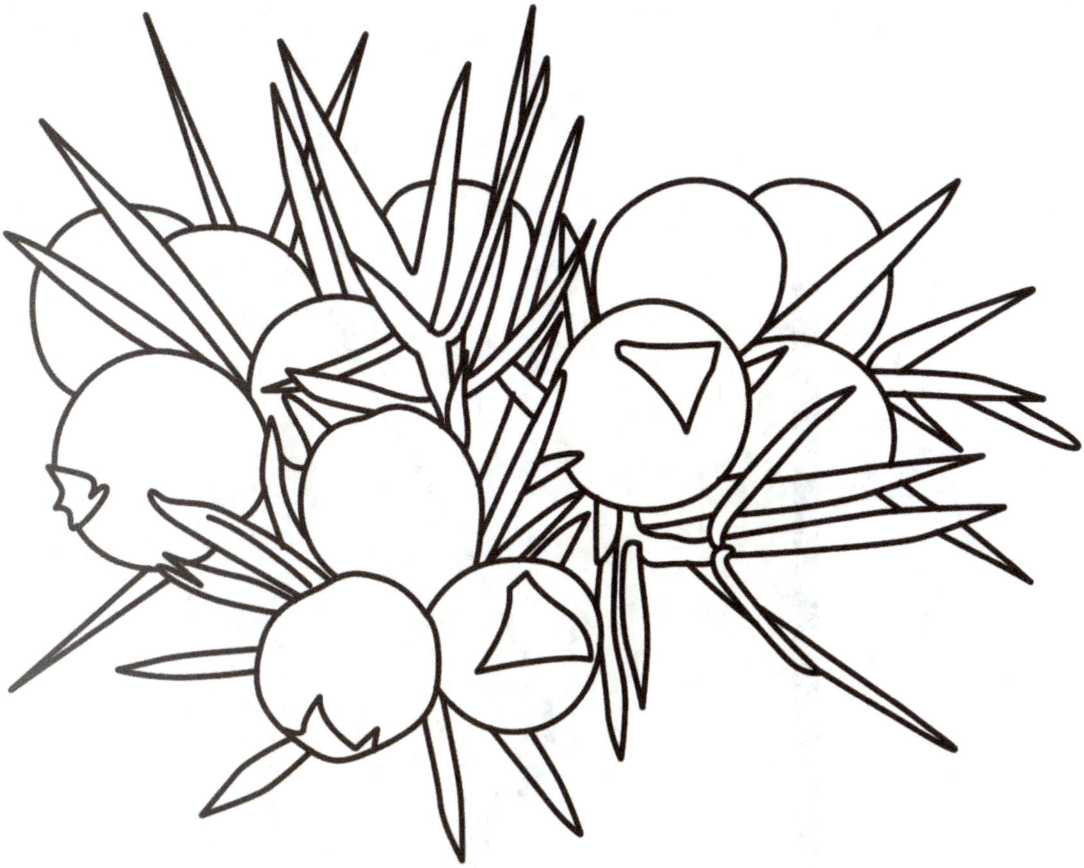

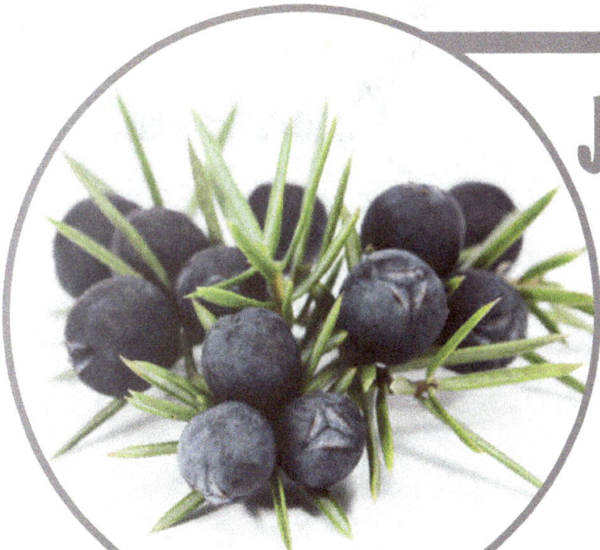

Juniper Berry

(joo•nuh•pr beh•ree)

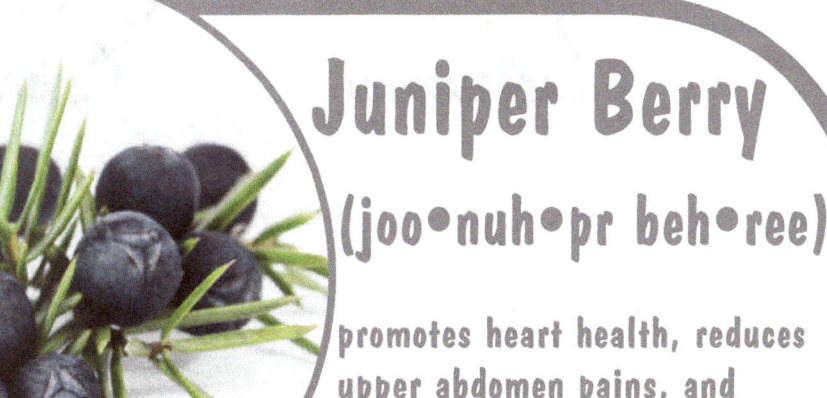

promotes heart health, reduces upper abdomen pains, and reduces inflammation

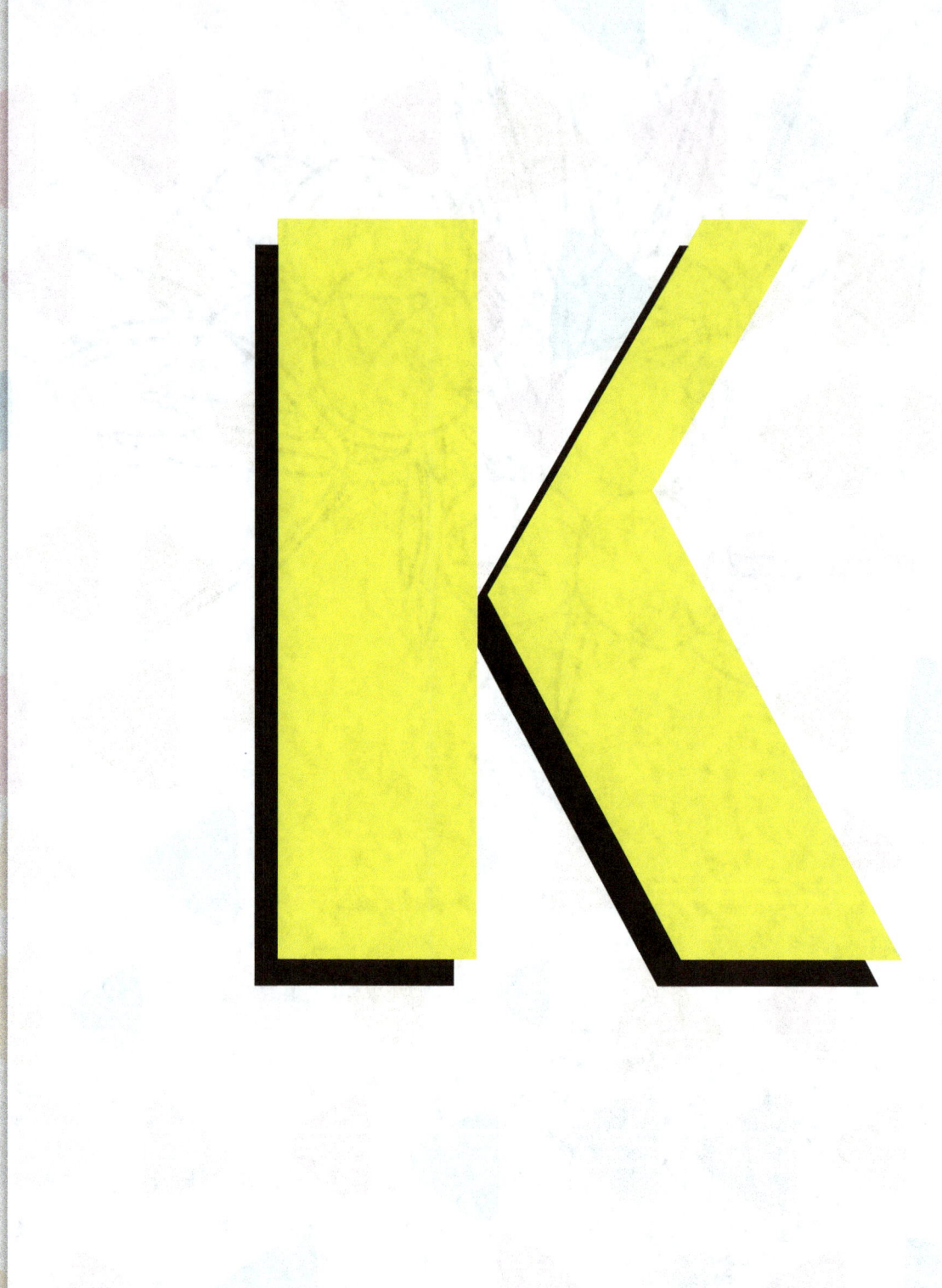

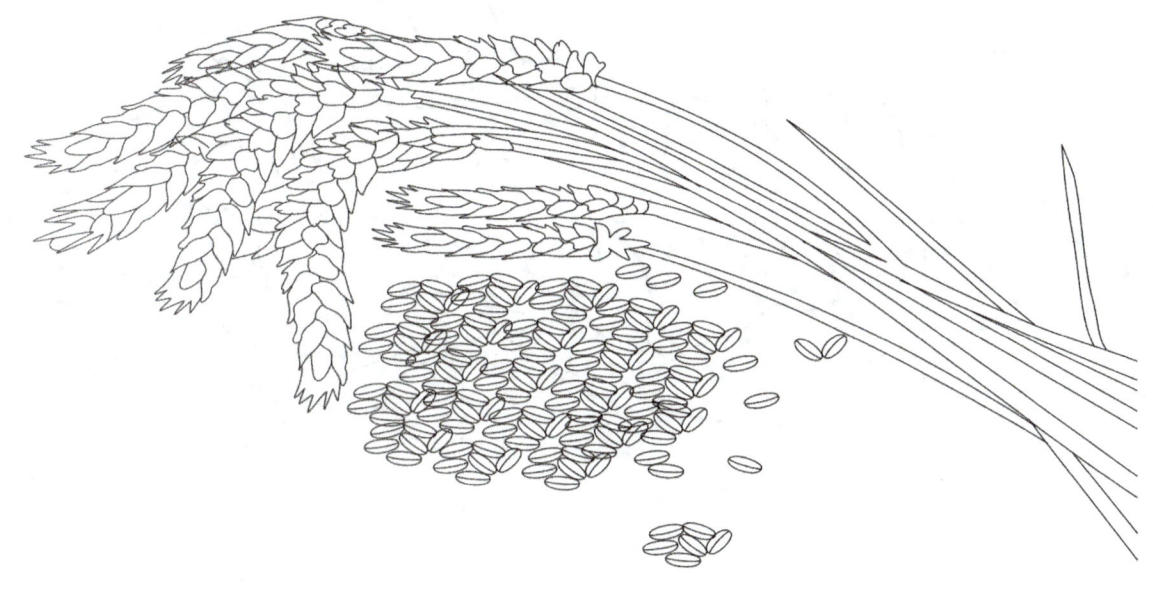

Kamut
(kah•moot)

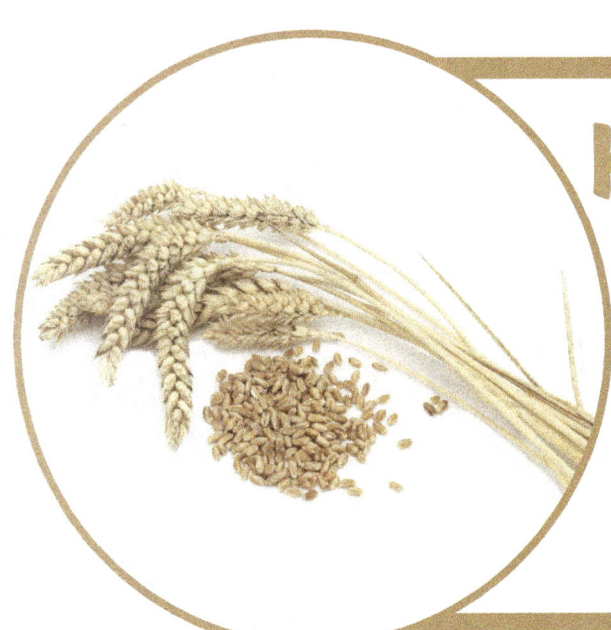

anti-inflammatory, supports bone health, and high in amino acids

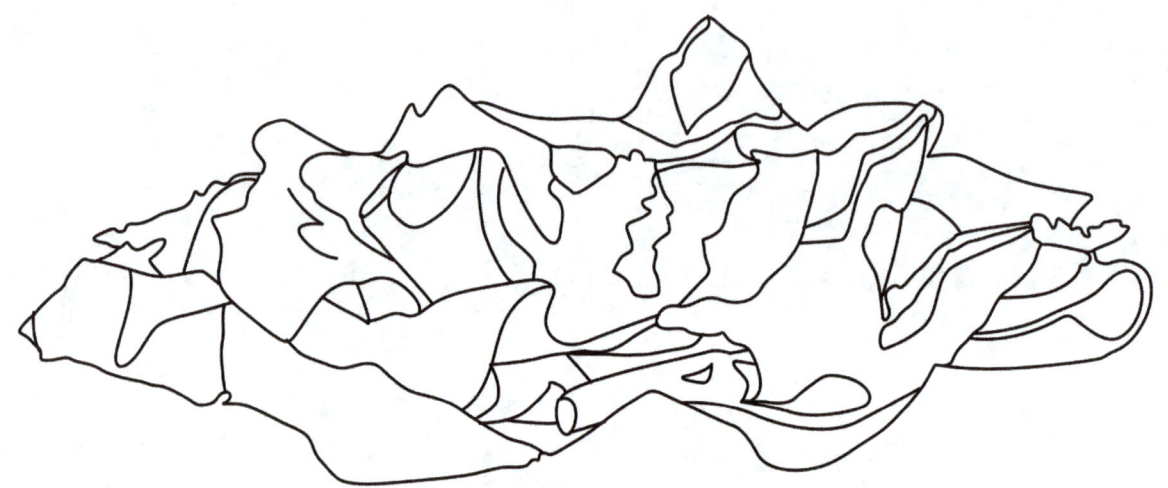

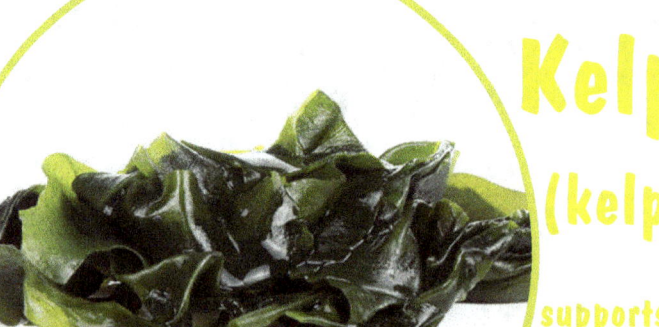

Kelp
(kelp)

supports cardiovascular health, high in iron, and rich source of iodine which regulates hormones in the body

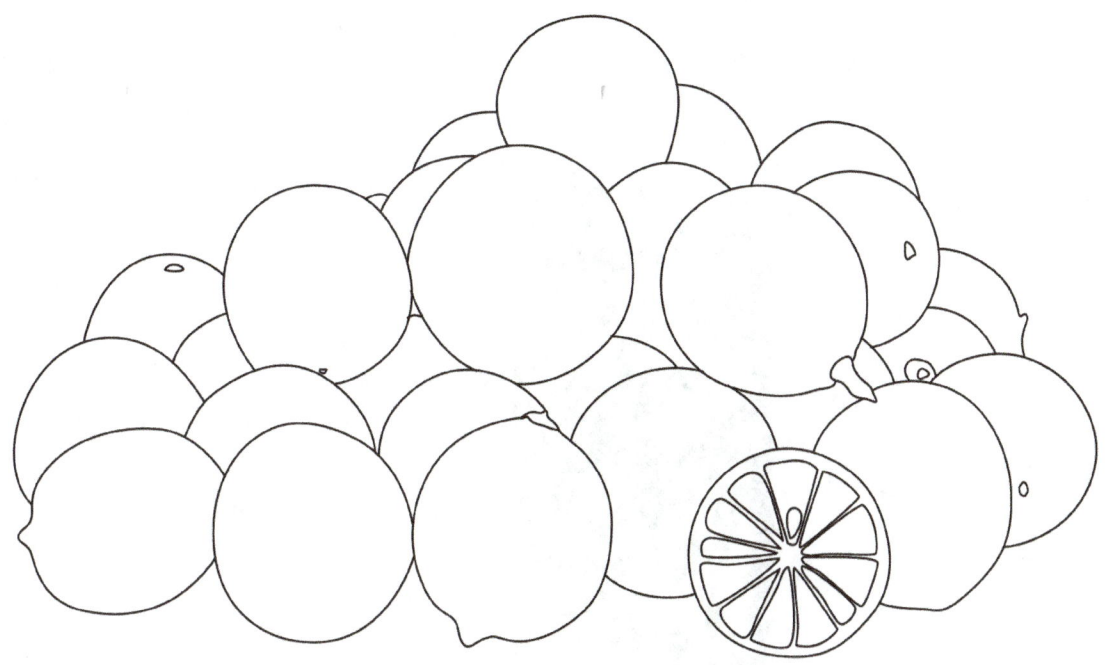

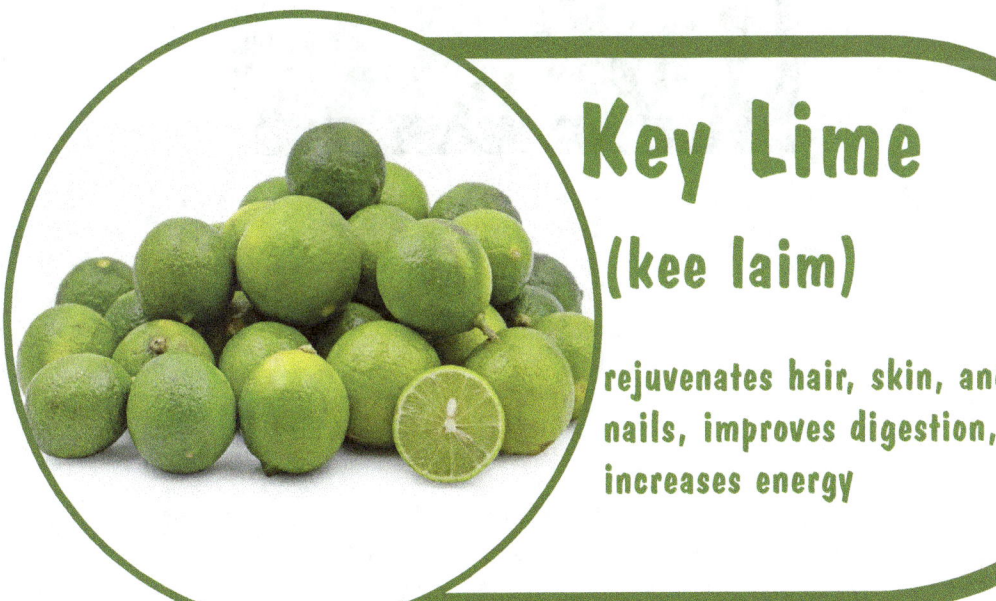

Key Lime

(kee laim)

rejuvenates hair, skin, and nails, improves digestion, and increases energy

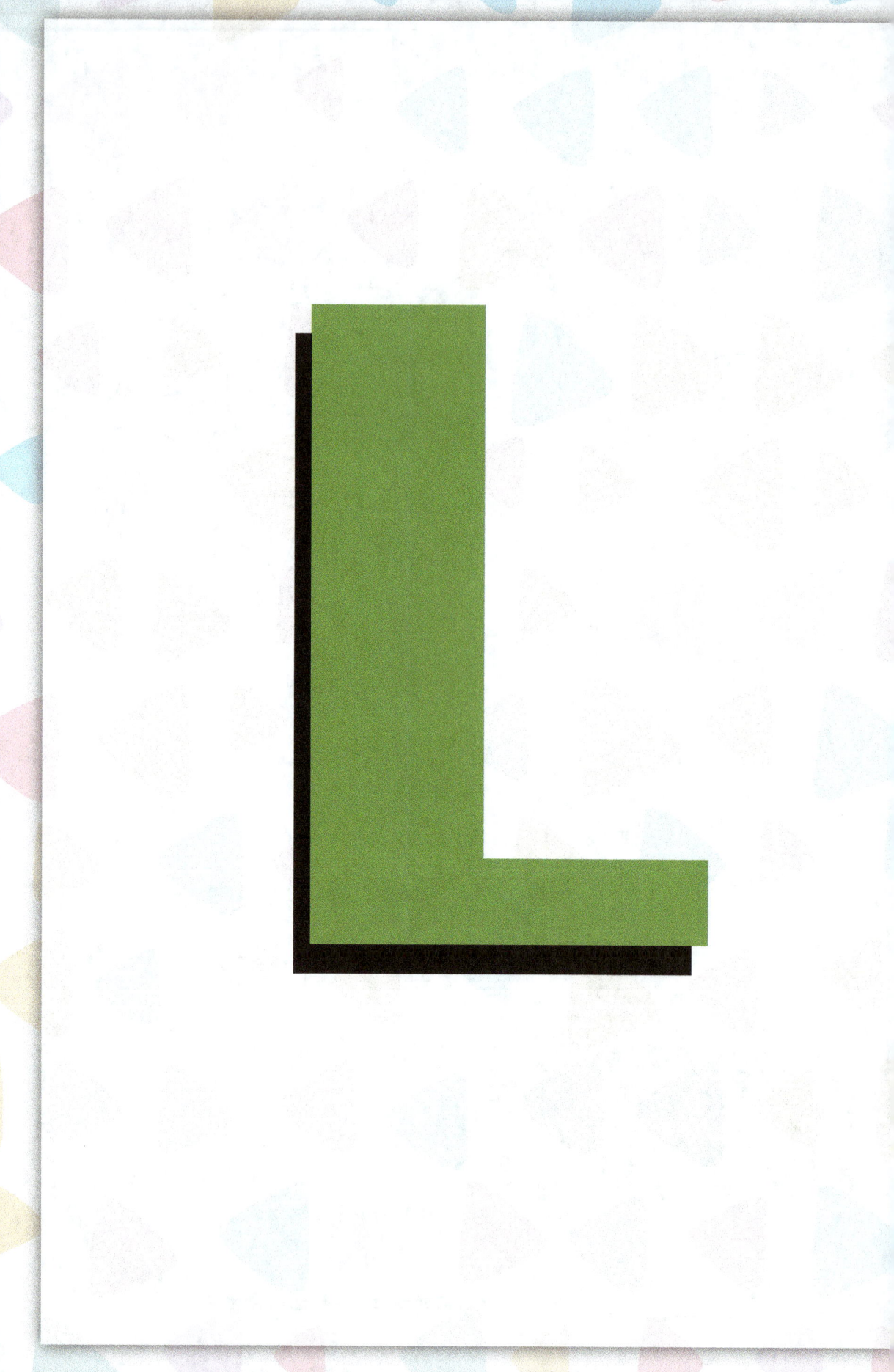

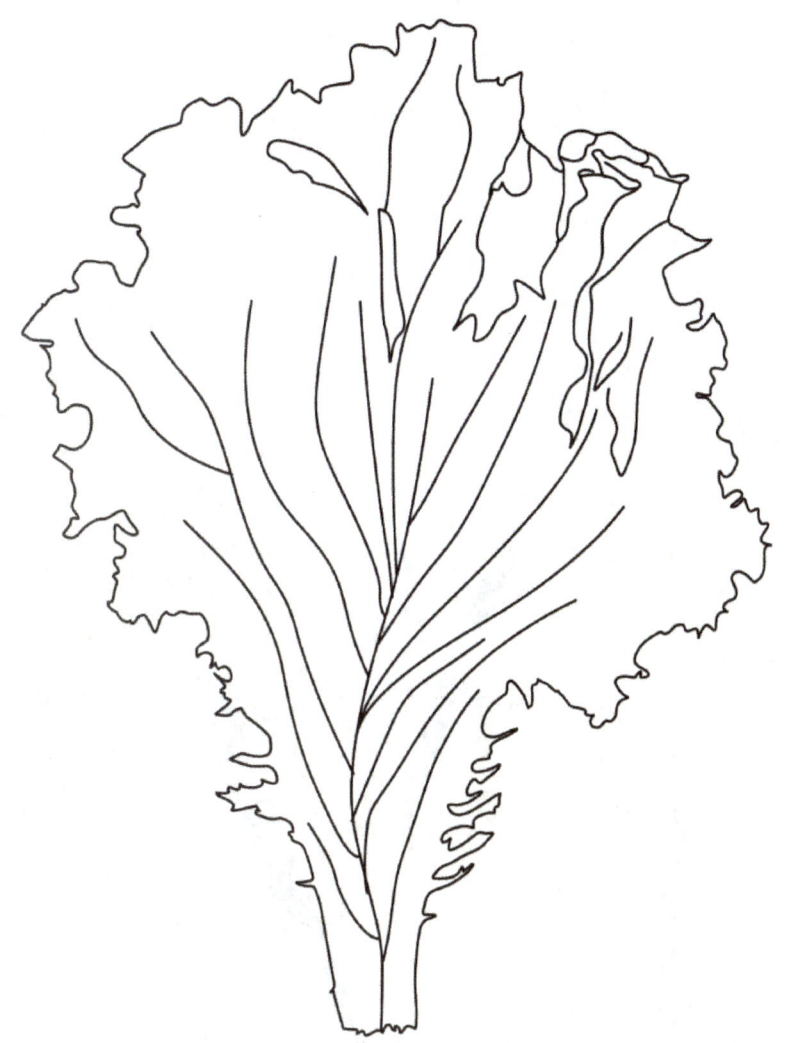

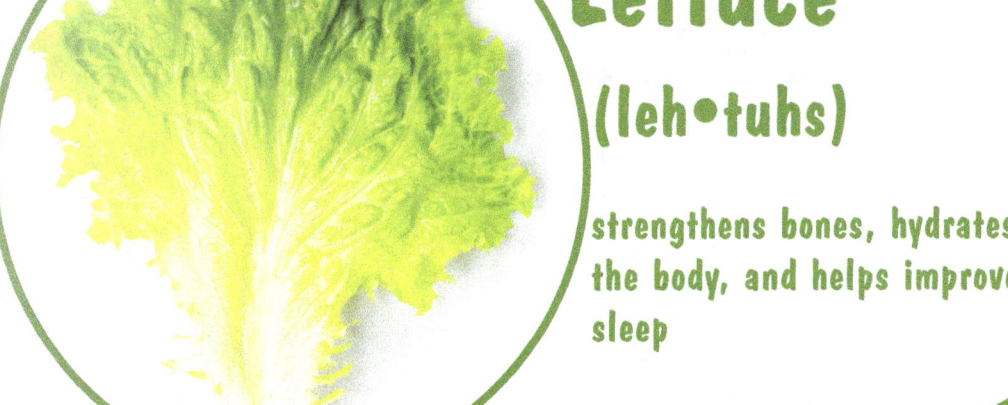

Lettuce
(leh•tuhs)

strengthens bones, hydrates the body, and helps improve sleep

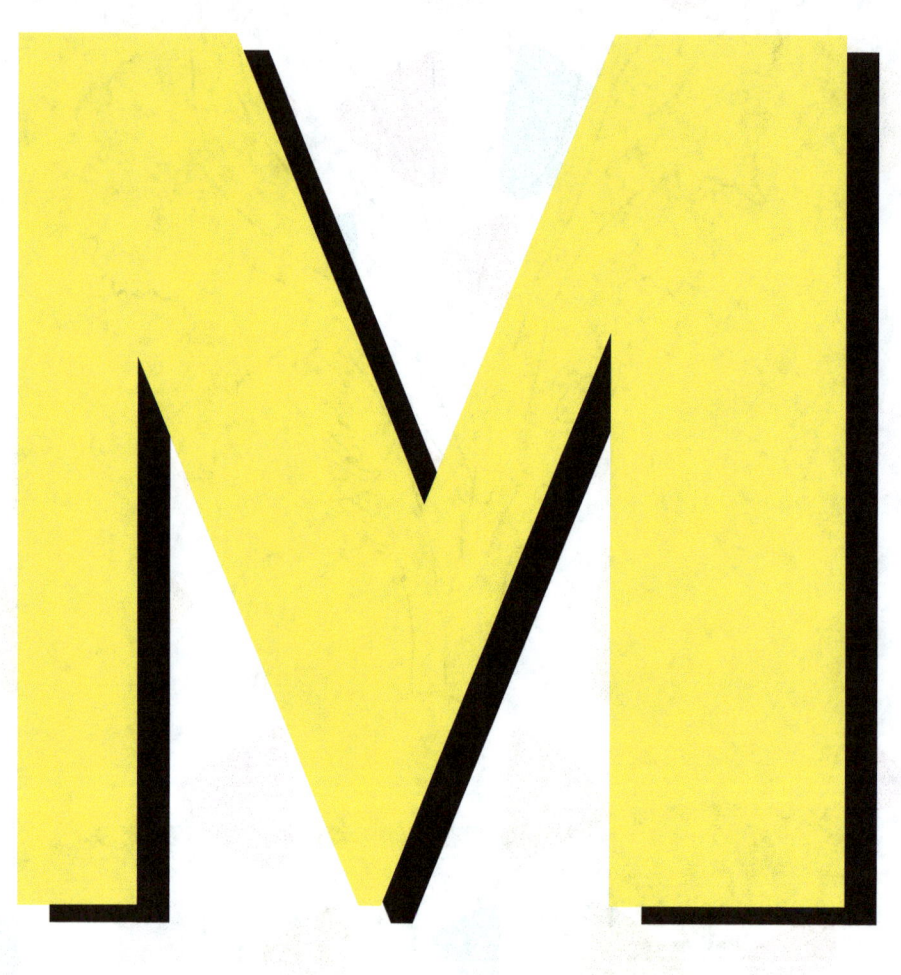

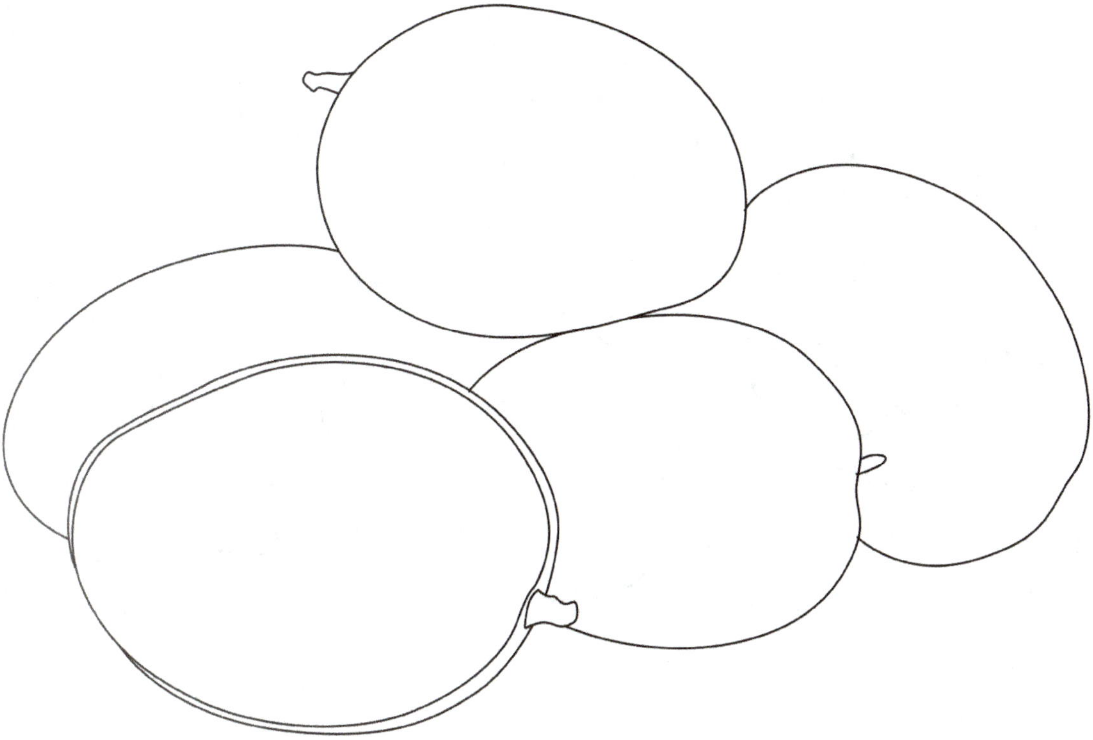

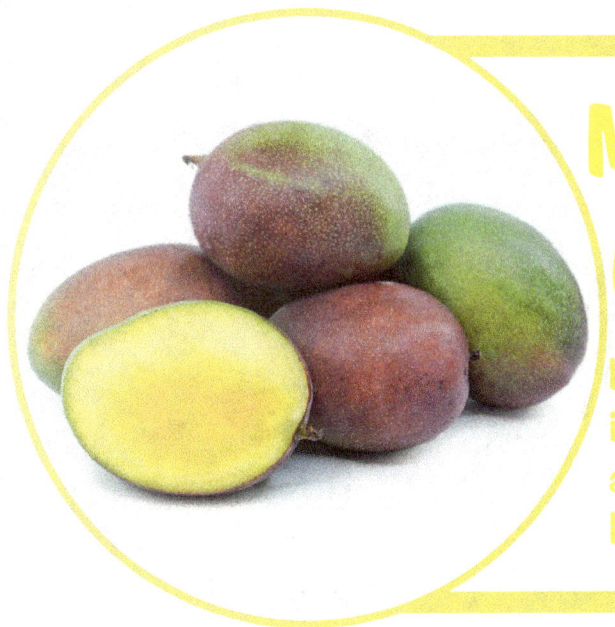

Mango
(mang•gow)

hydrates the body, boosts immunity, supports heart health, and promotes skin and hair health

65

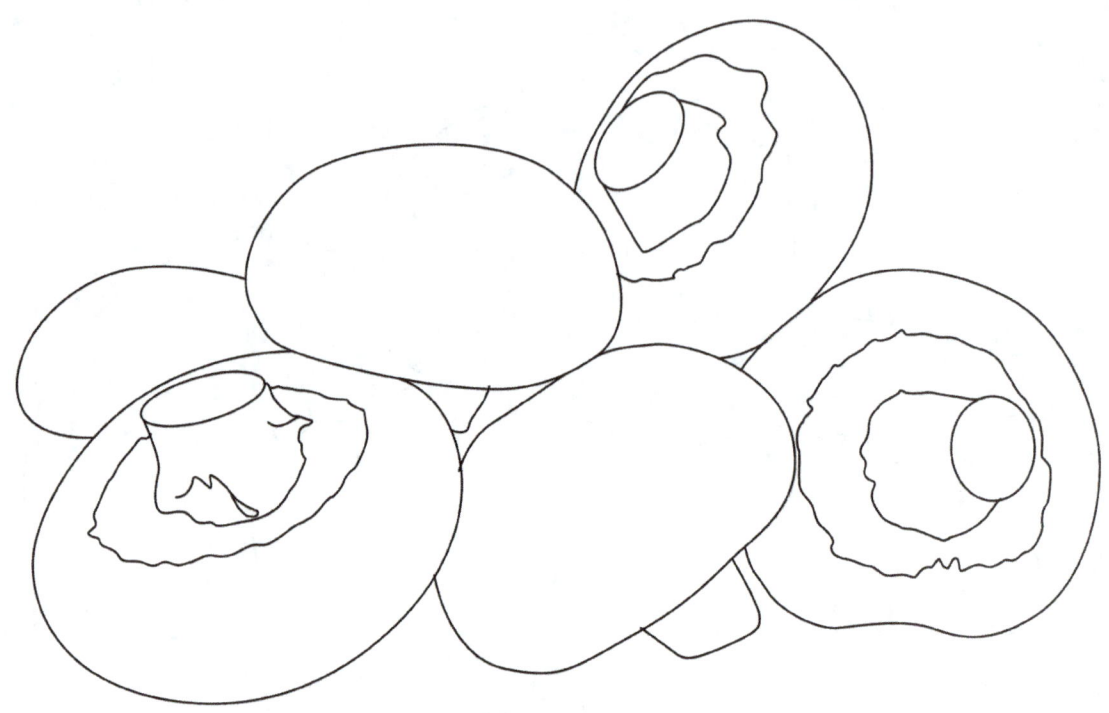

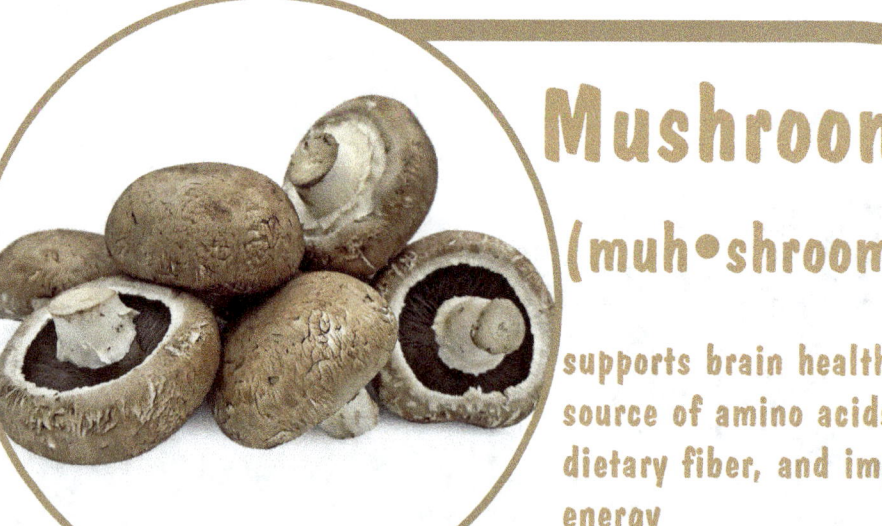

Mushrooms
(muh•shroomz)

supports brain health, good source of amino acids and dietary fiber, and improves energy

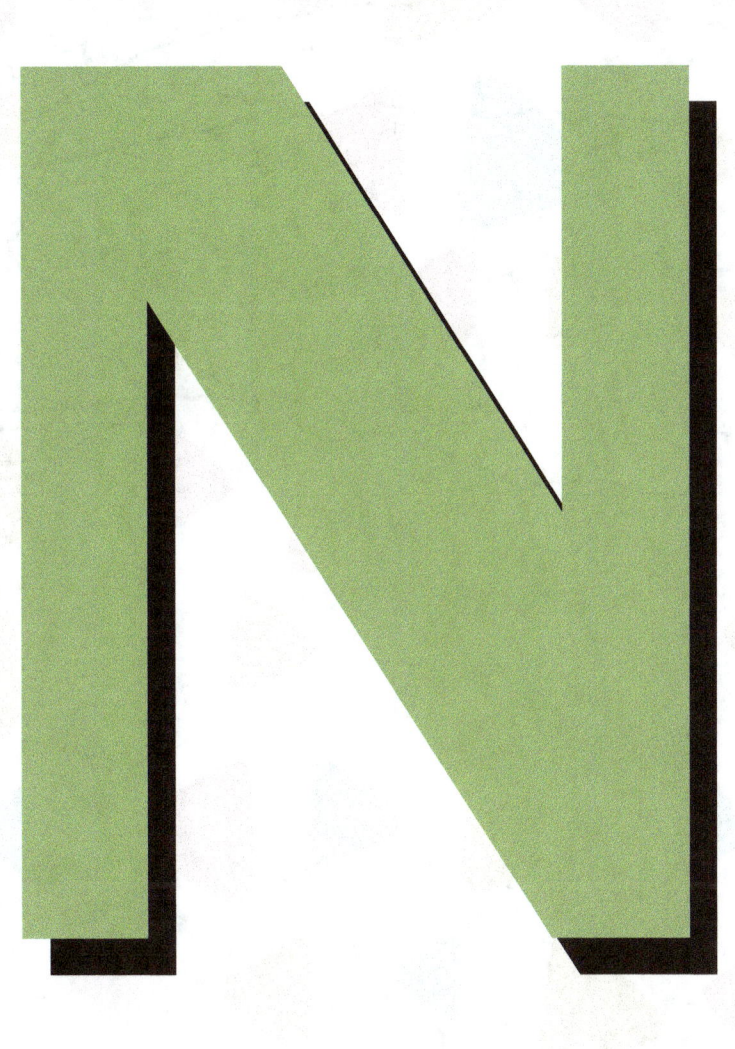

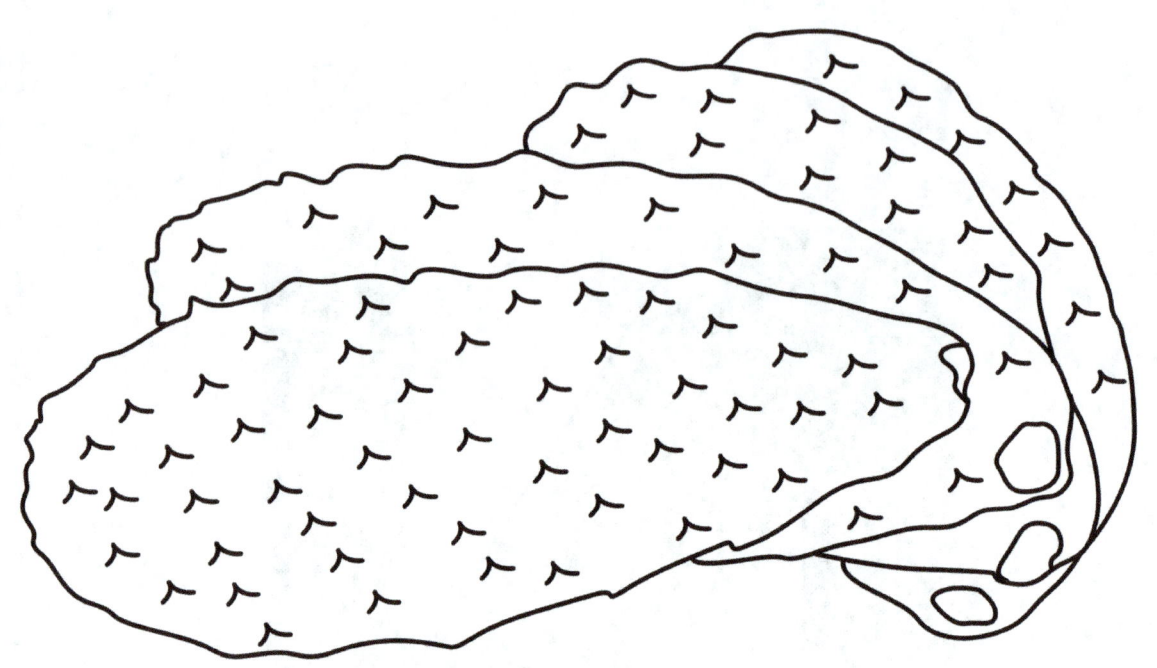

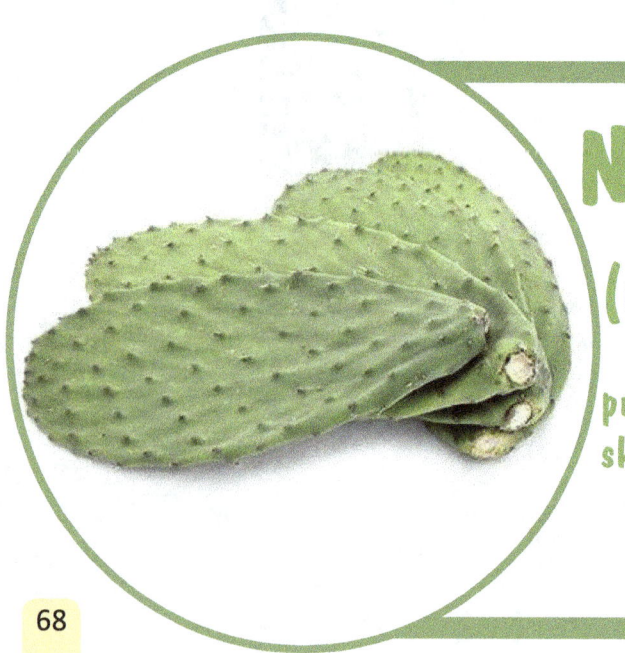

Nopal
(no•paal)

protects nerves, hydrates the skin, and supports heart health

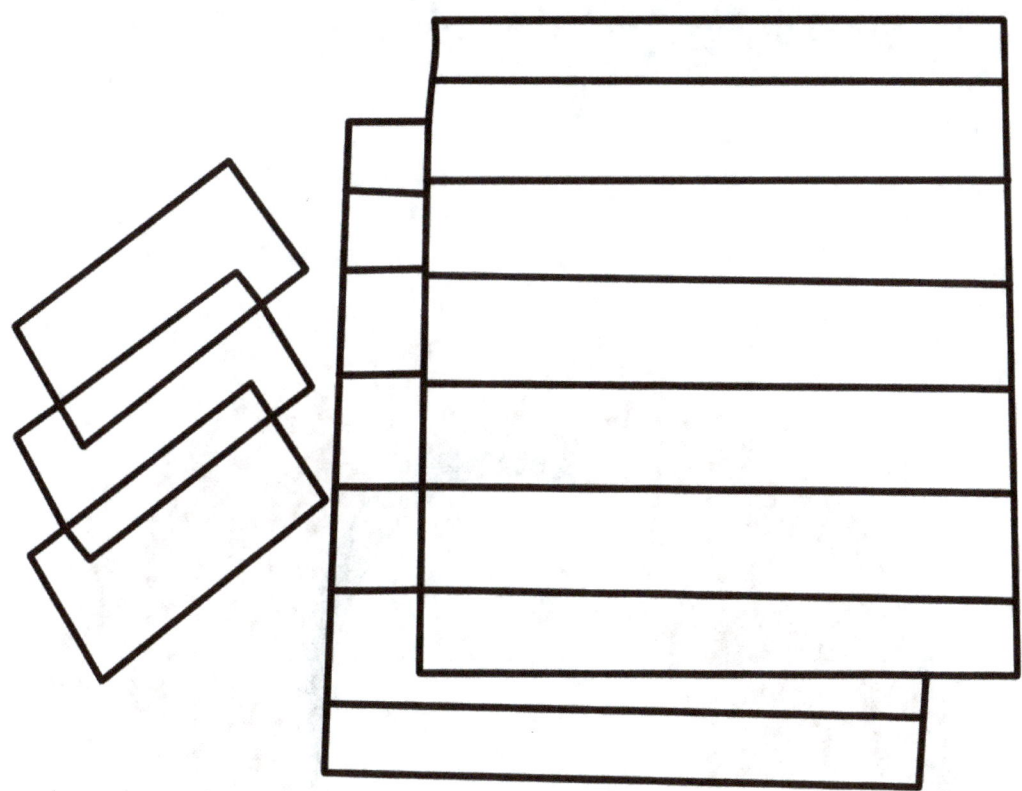

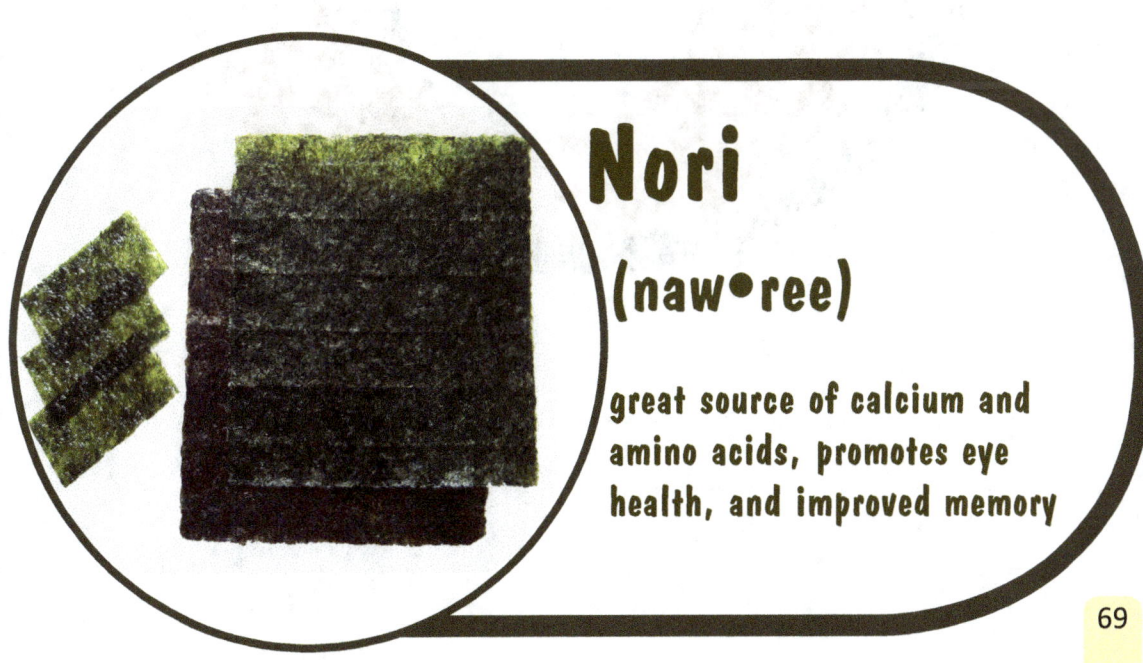

Nori

(naw•ree)

great source of calcium and amino acids, promotes eye health, and improved memory

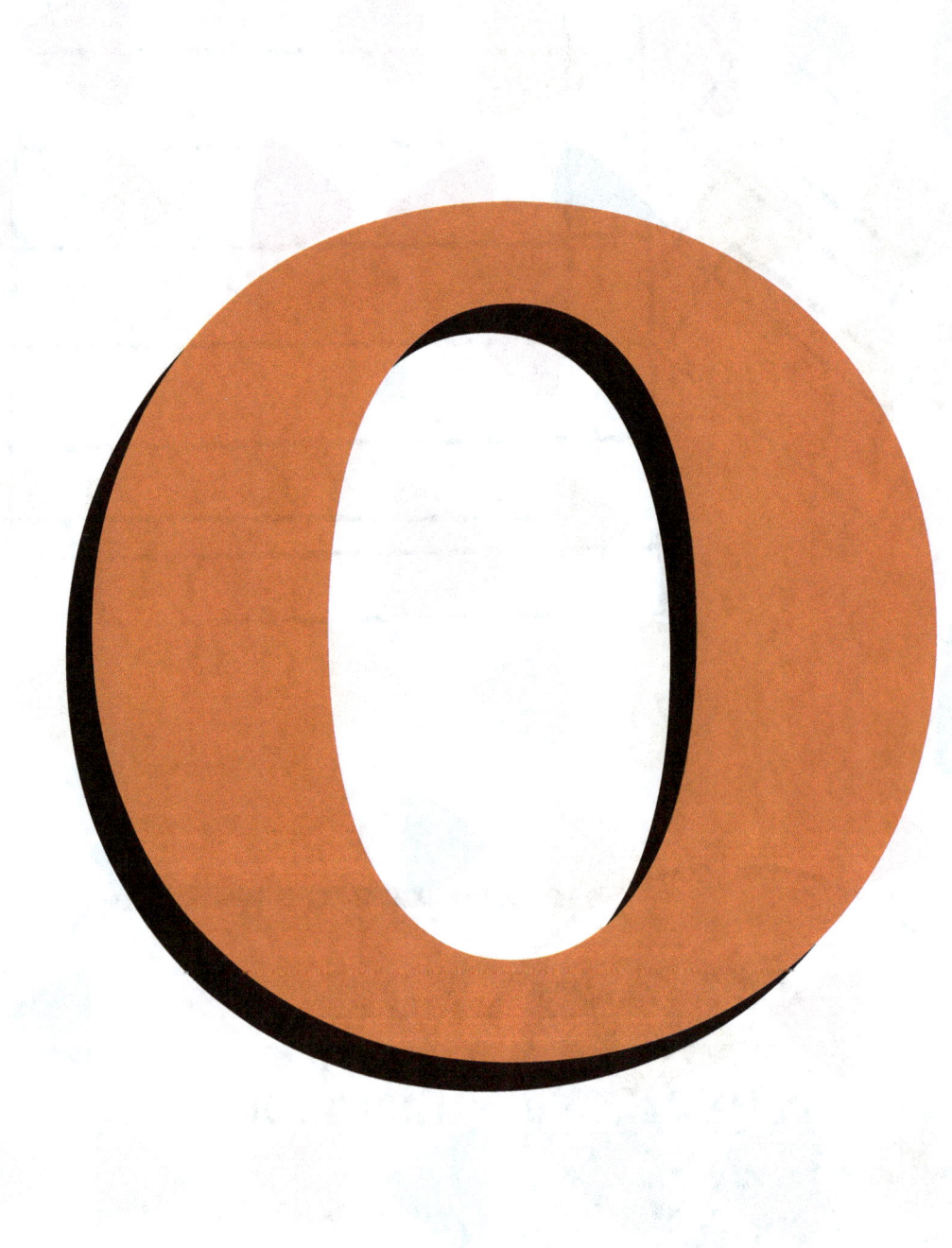

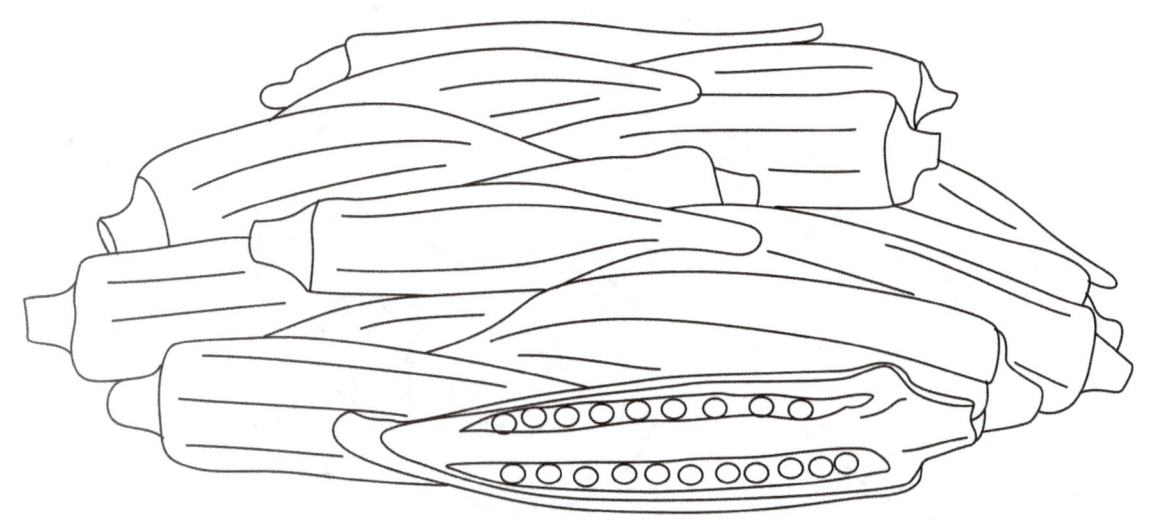

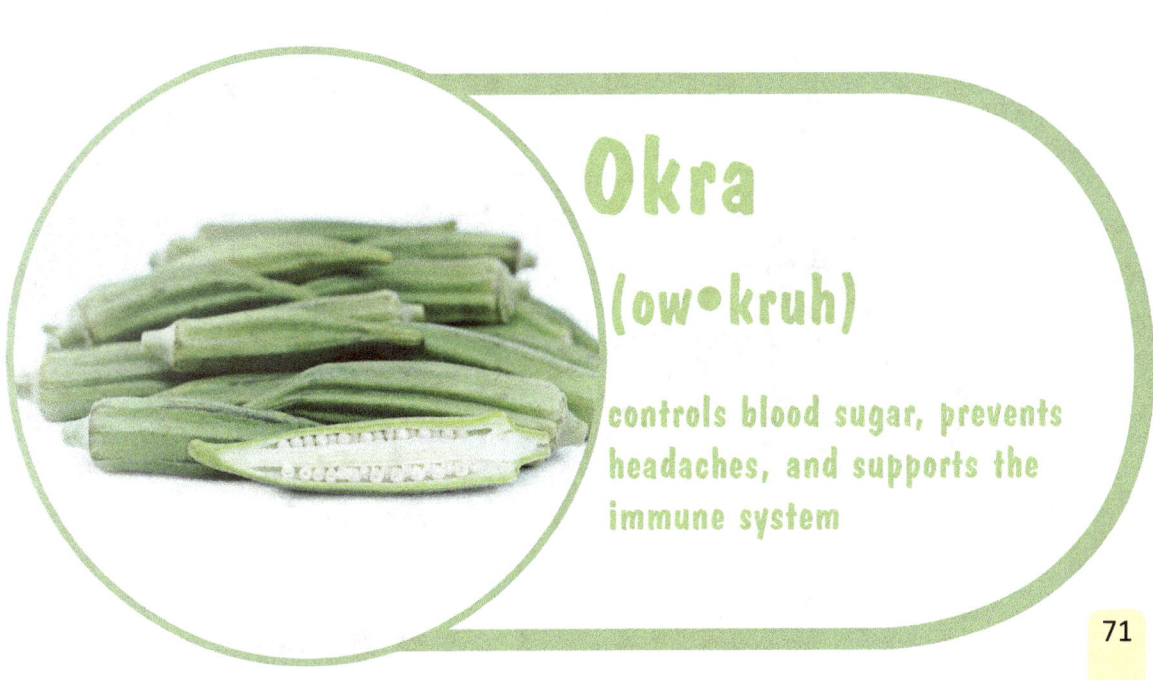

Okra
(ow•kruh)

controls blood sugar, prevents headaches, and supports the immune system

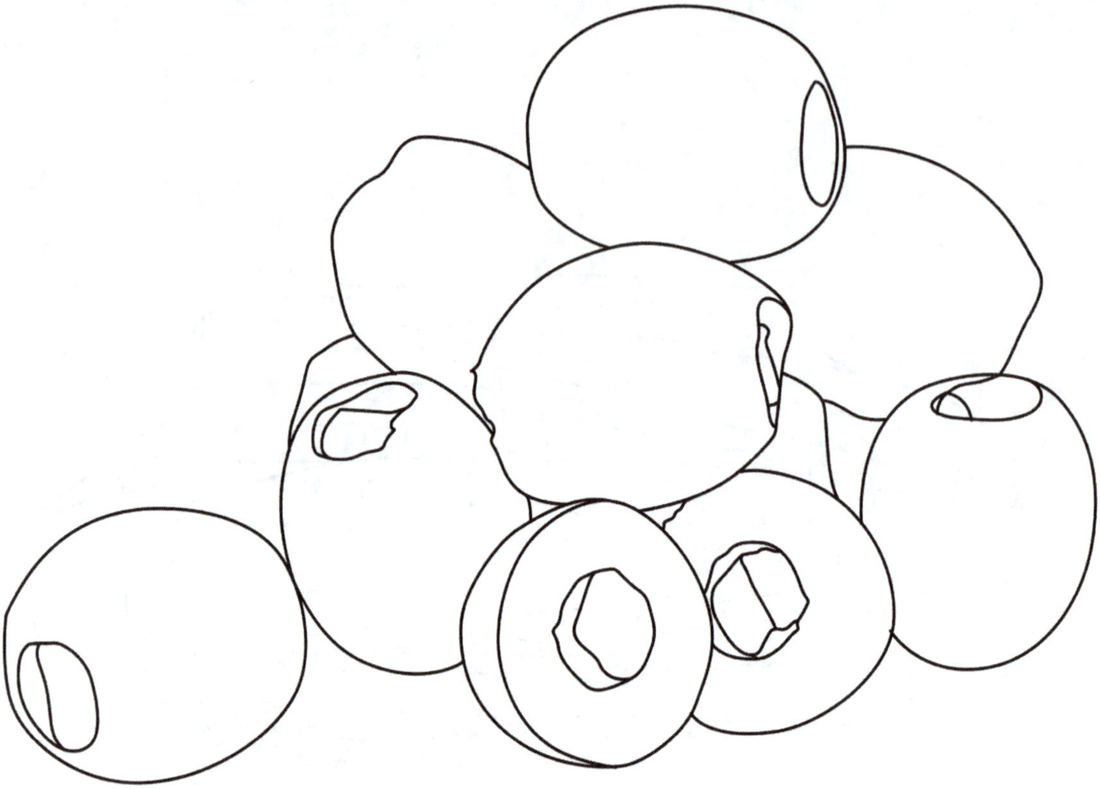

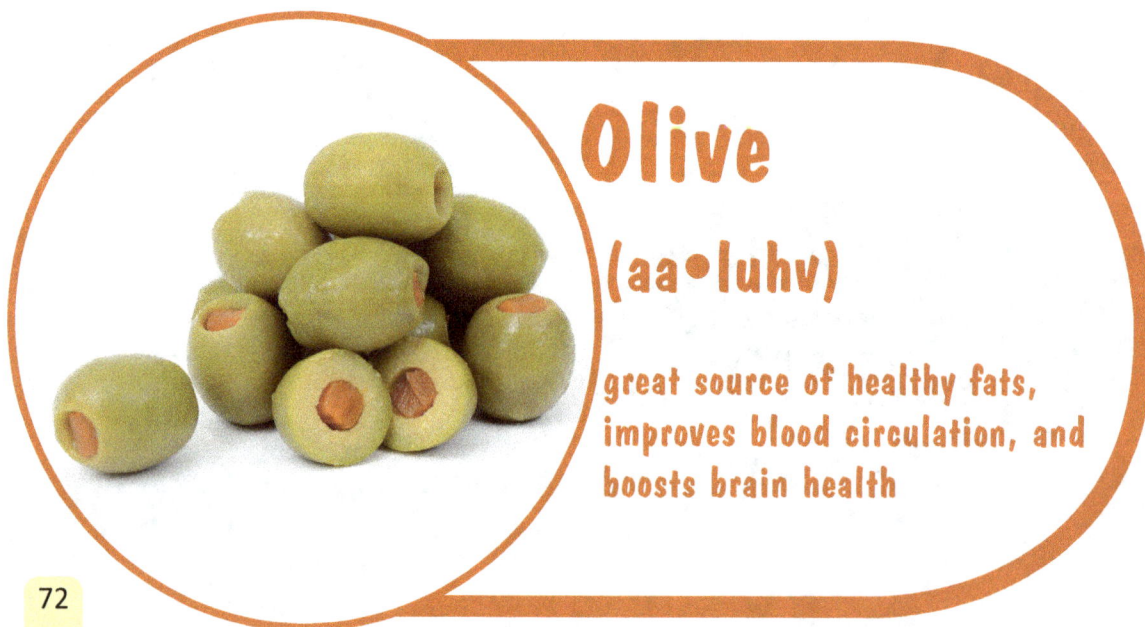

Olive
(aa•luhv)

great source of healthy fats, improves blood circulation, and boosts brain health

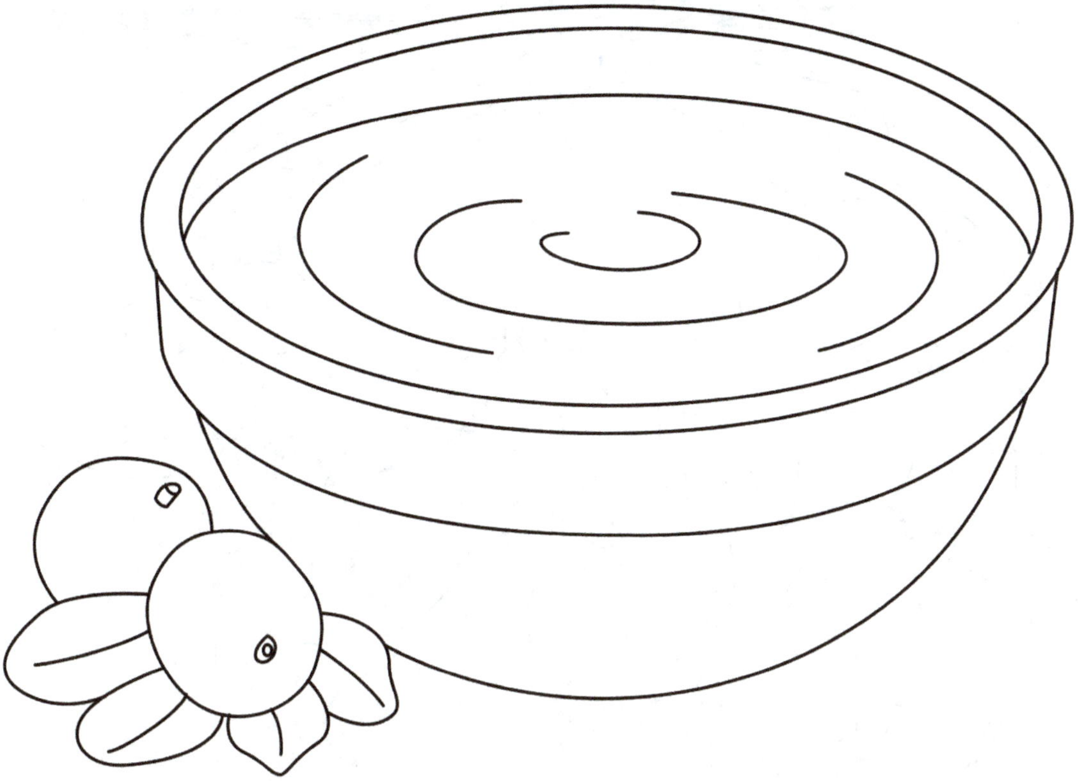

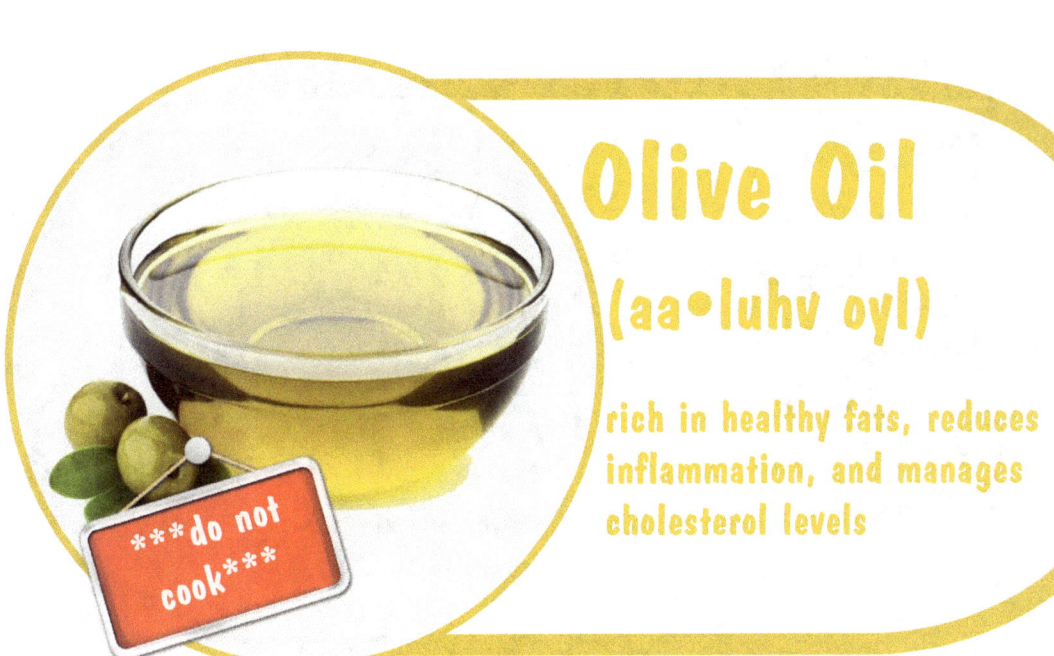

Olive Oil
(aa•luhv oyl)

rich in healthy fats, reduces inflammation, and manages cholesterol levels

do not cook

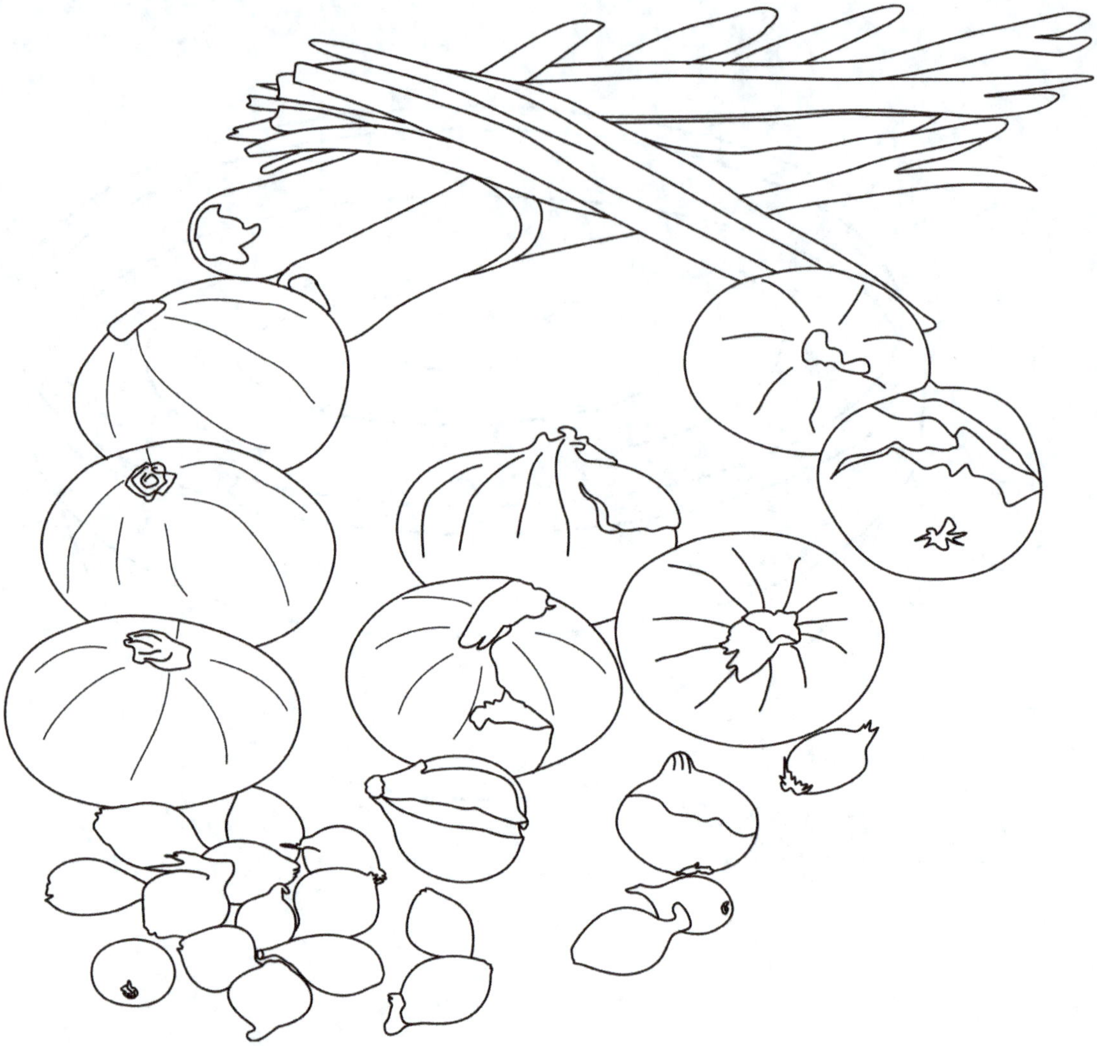

Onion
(uhn•yn)

lowers risk of heart disease, improves bone health, and promotes healthy skin, hair, and nails

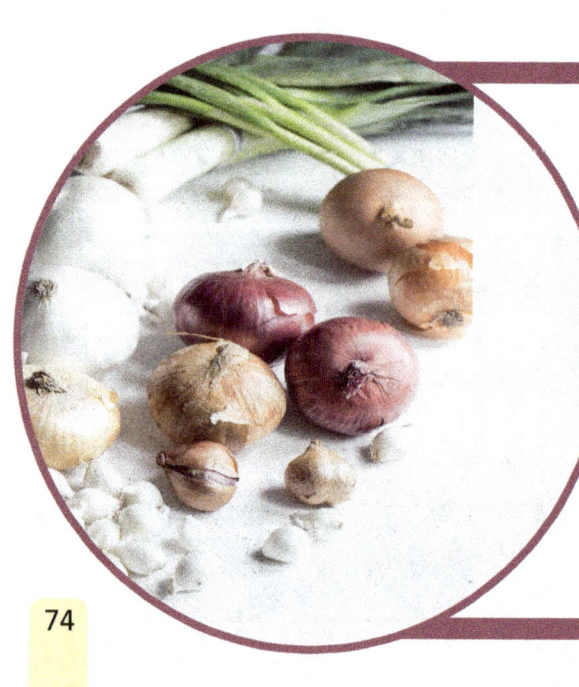

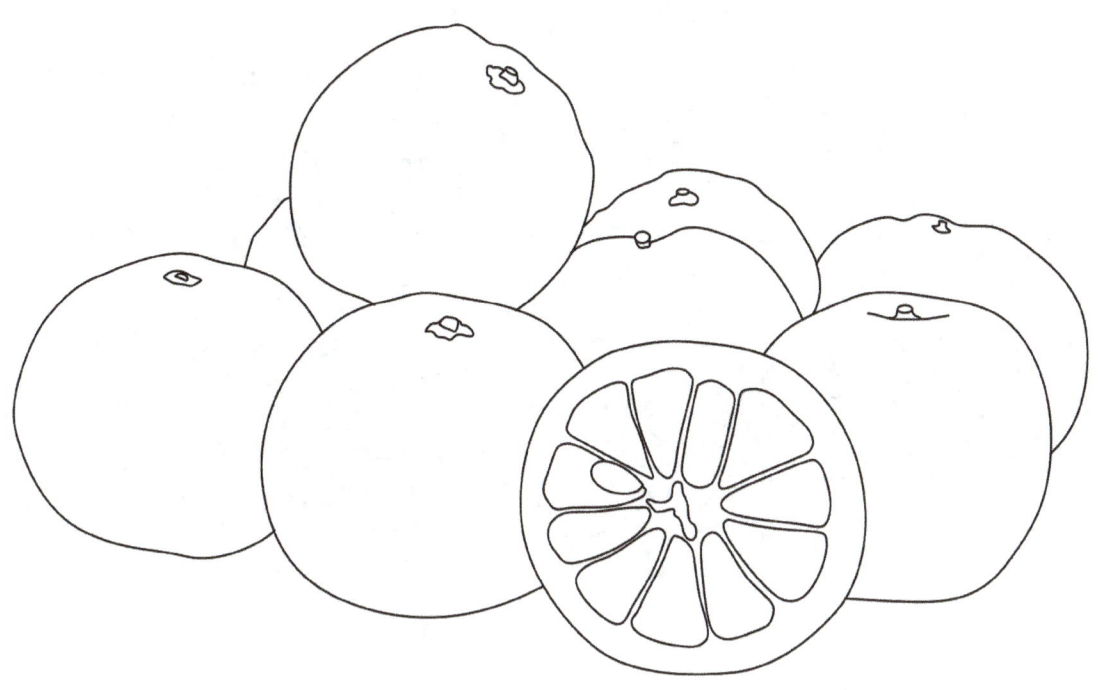

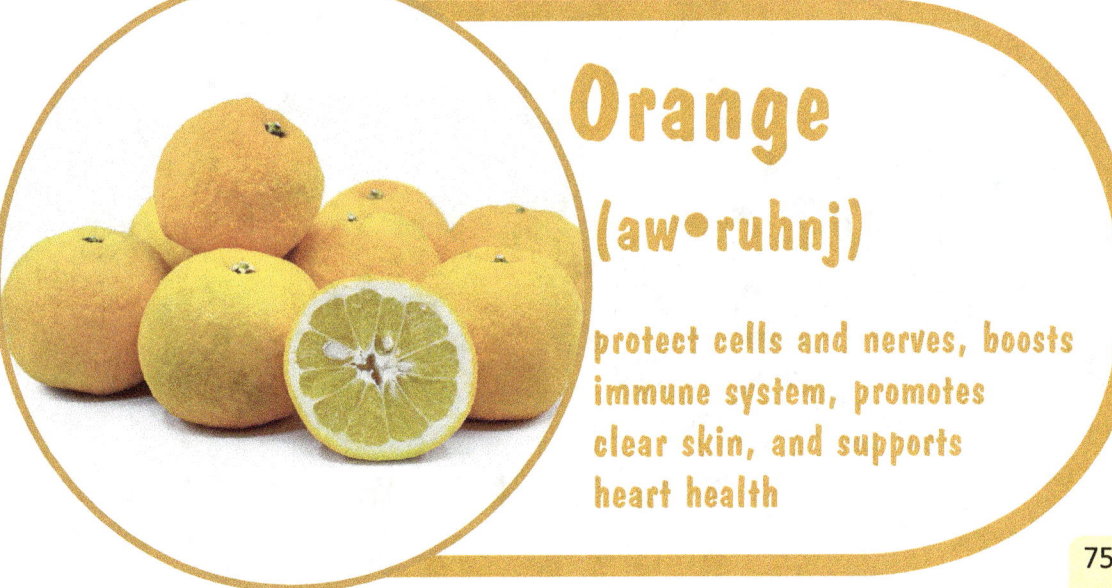

Orange
(aw•ruhnj)

protect cells and nerves, boosts immune system, promotes clear skin, and supports heart health

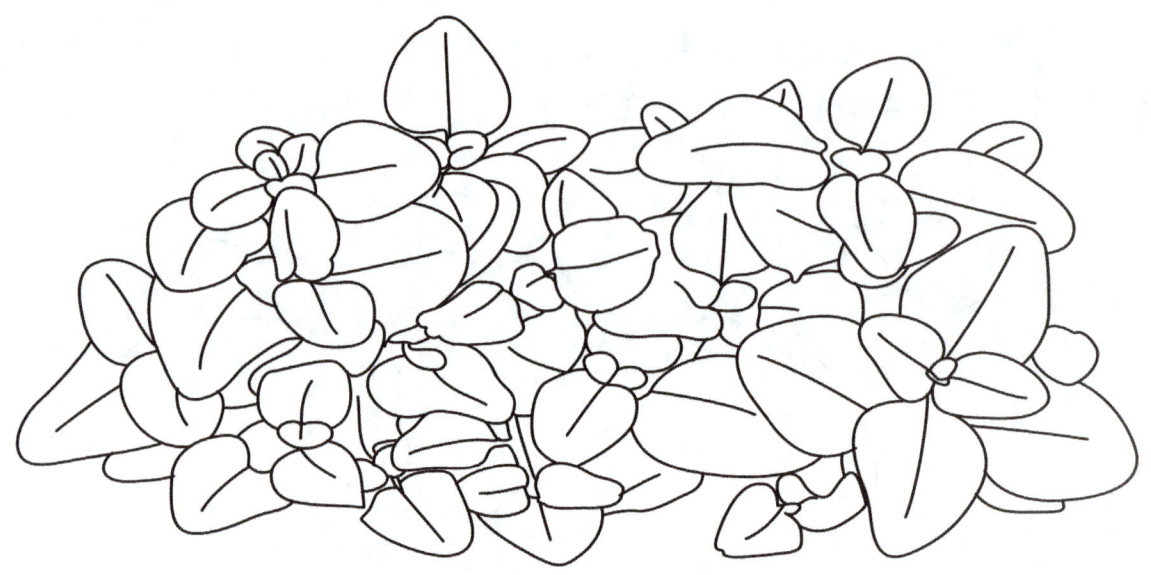

Oregano
(uh•reh•guh•now)

prevents infections, repairs damaged cells, boosts immune system, helps soothe cough and sore throat

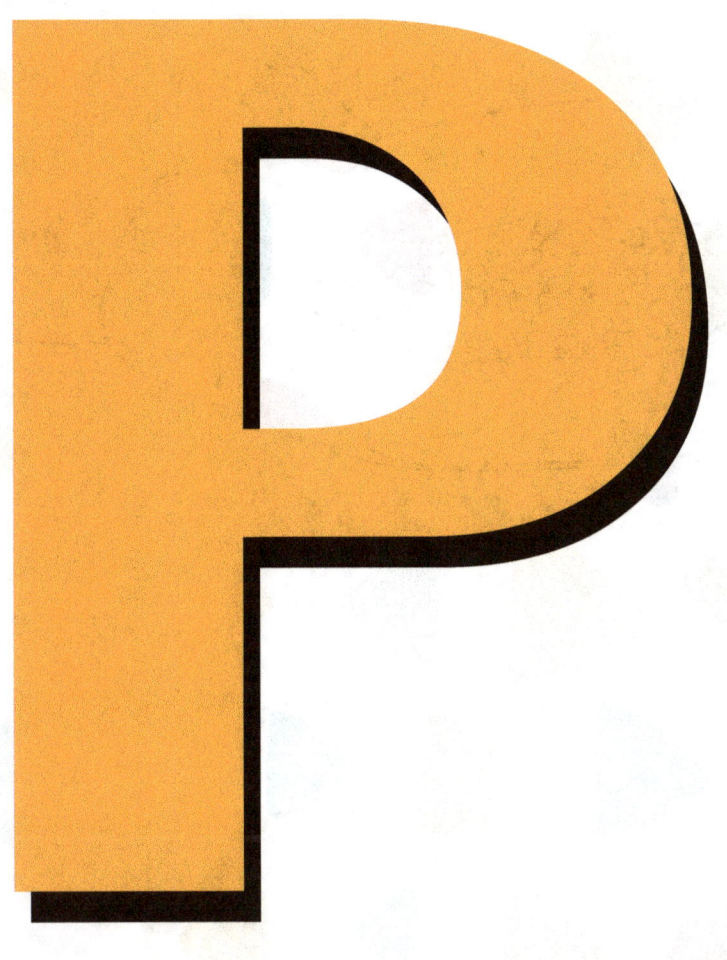

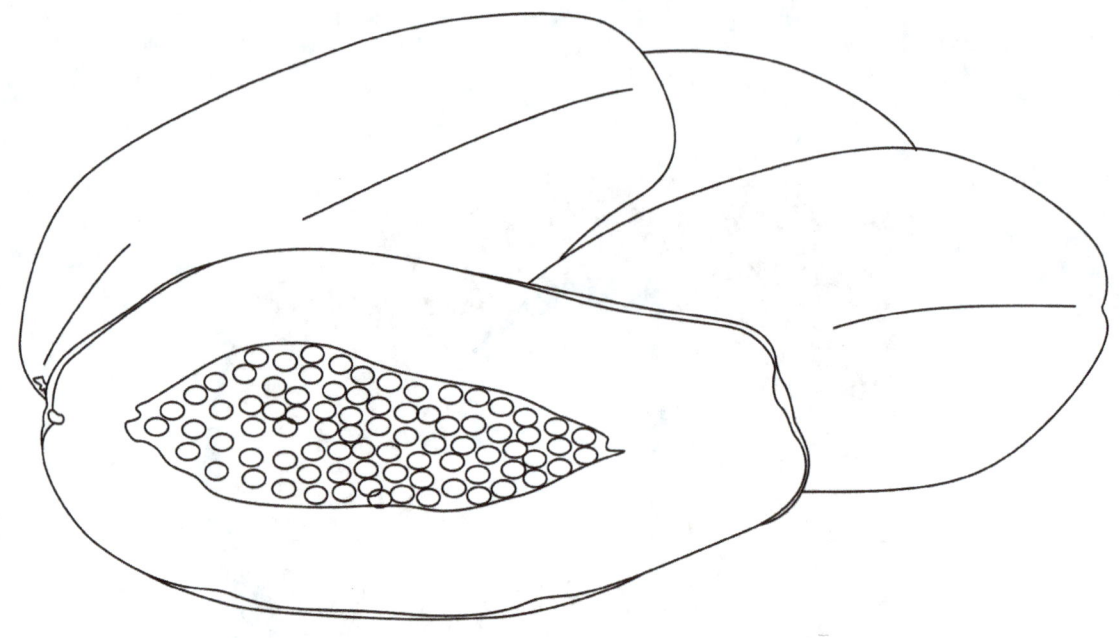

Papaya
(puh•pai•uh)

reduce risk of heart disease, keeps skin hydrated, and keeps digestive tract healthy

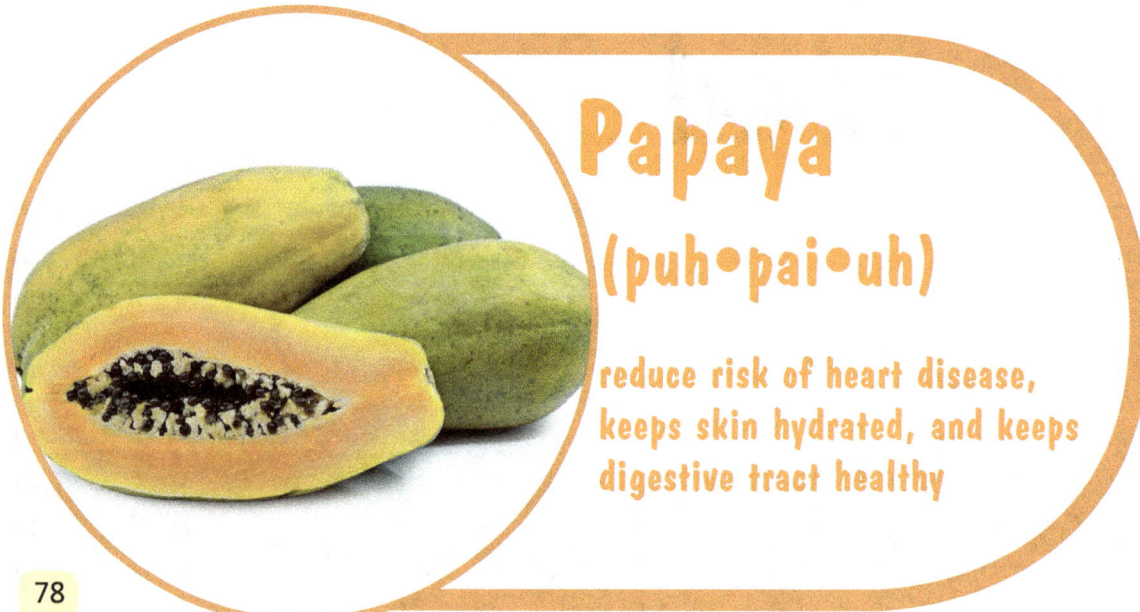

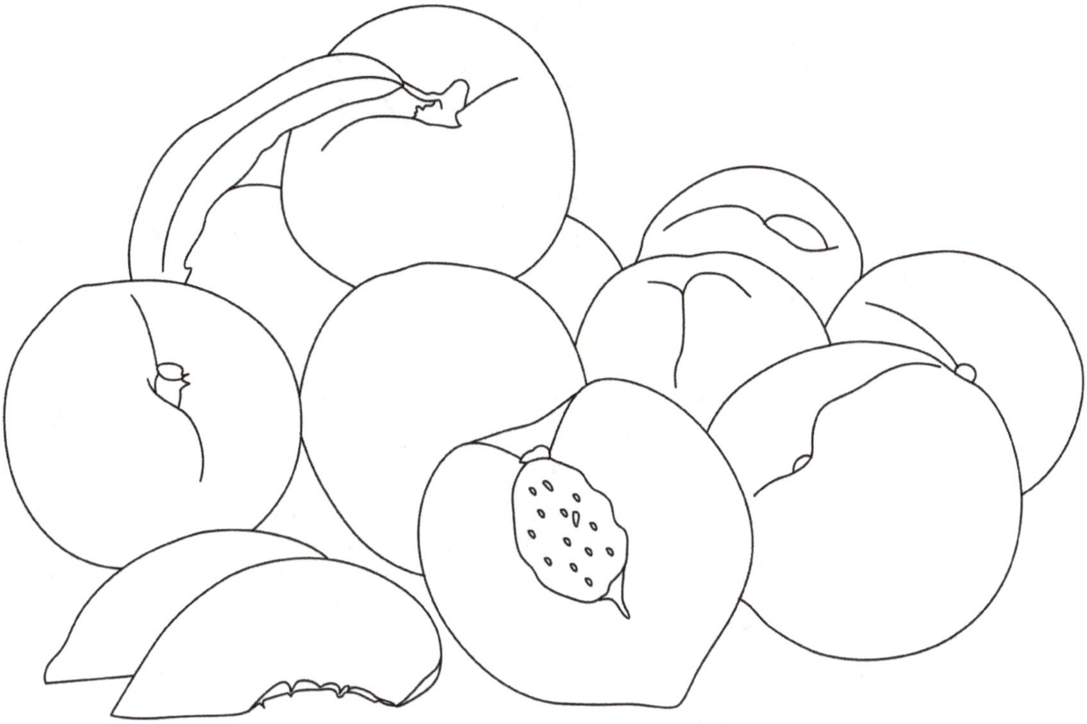

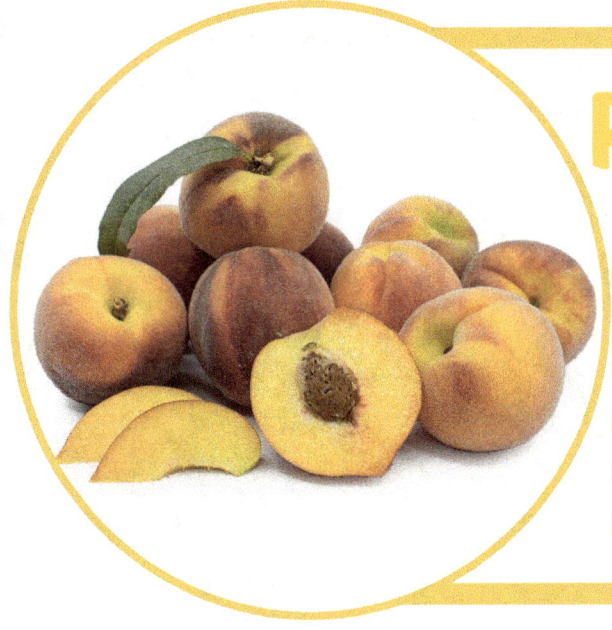

Peach
(peech)

regulates heart rate, protects the skin, reduces symptoms of allergies, helps remain hydrated, and promotes eye health

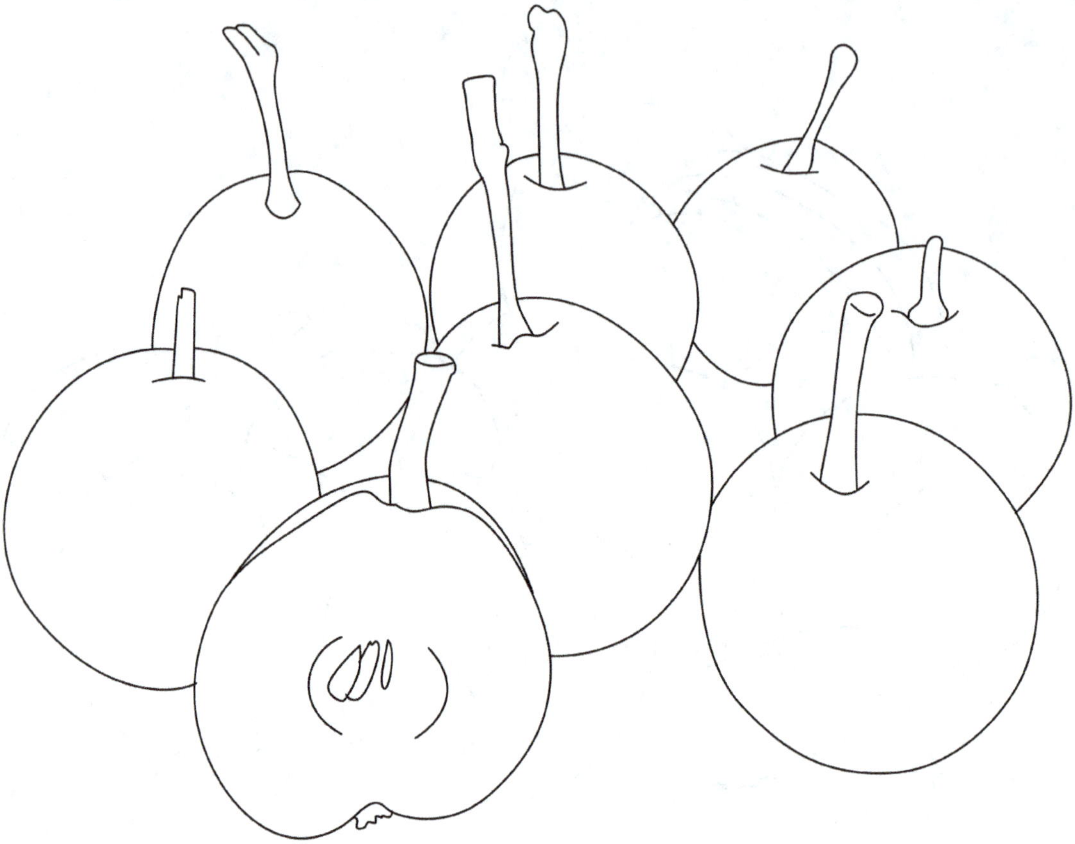

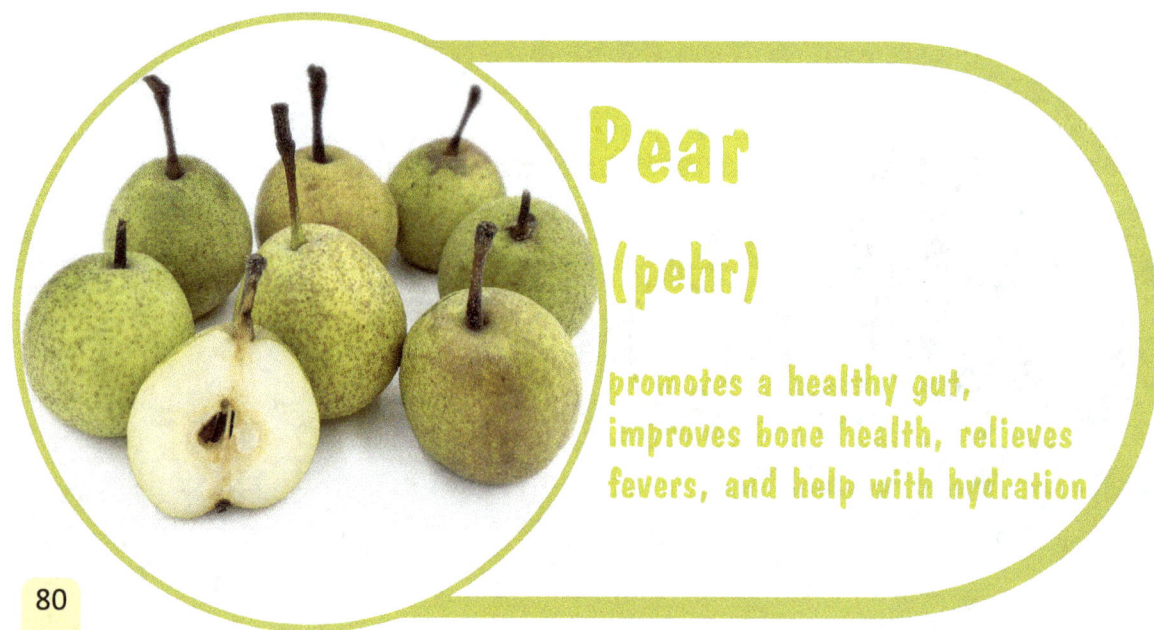

Pear
(pehr)

promotes a healthy gut, improves bone health, relieves fevers, and help with hydration

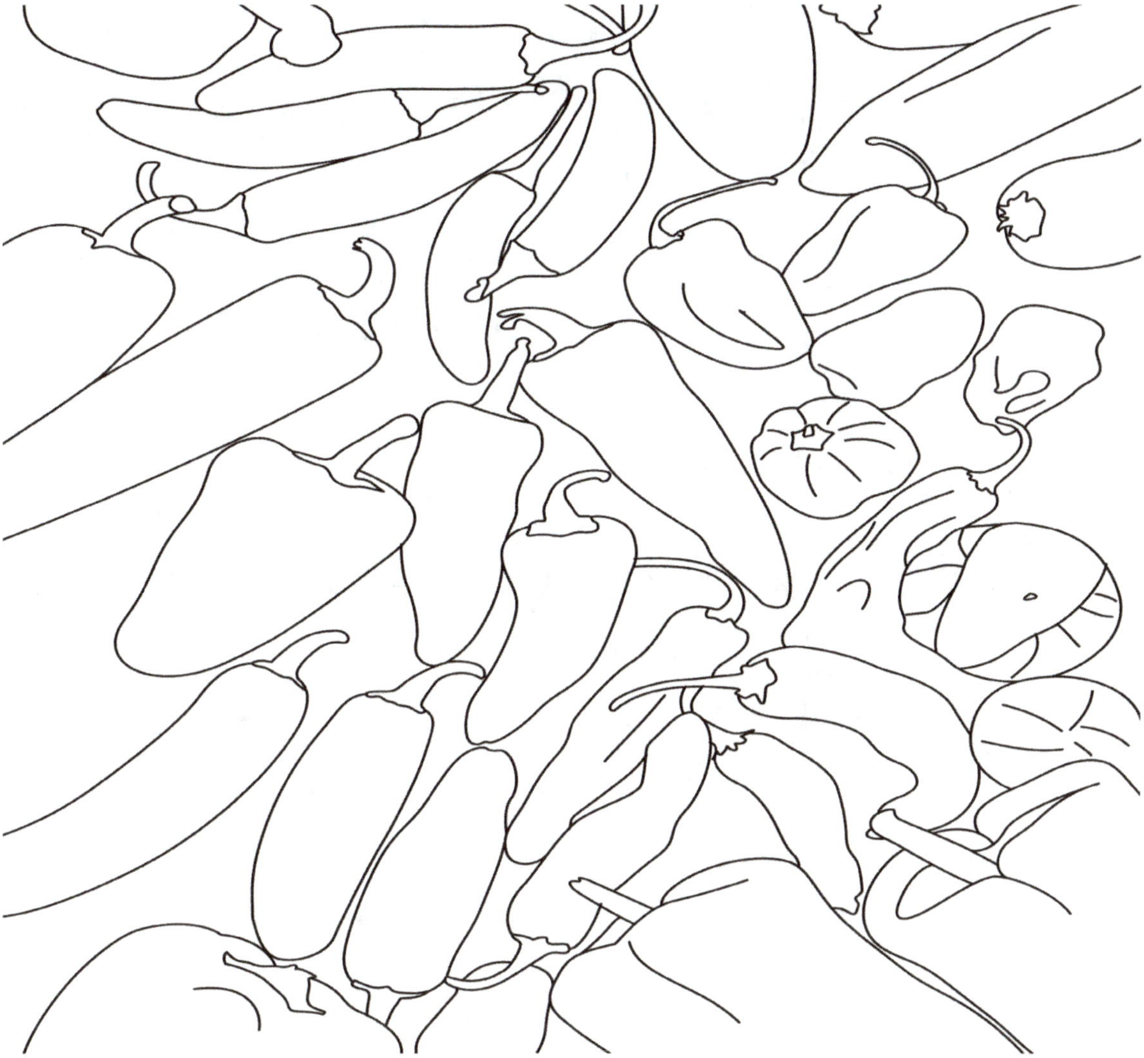

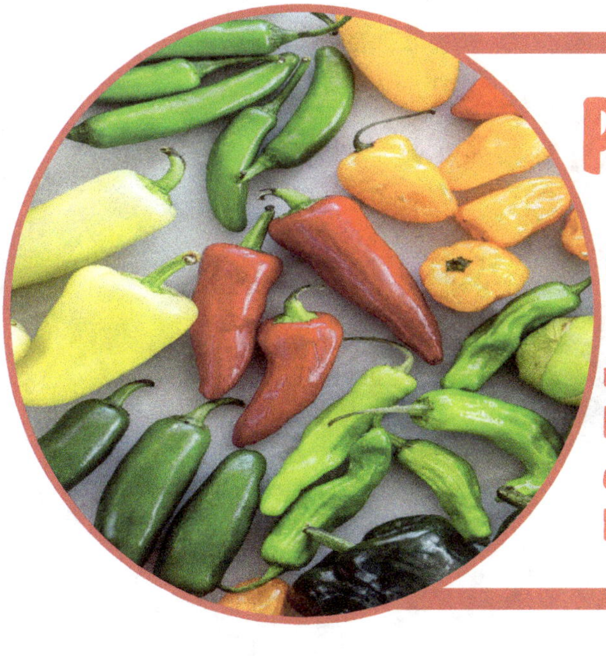

Pepper
(peh•pr)

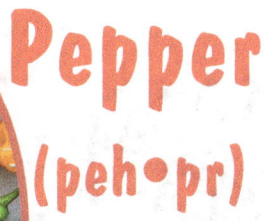

repairs damaged blood cells, keeps stomach and intestines clean, and promotes heart health

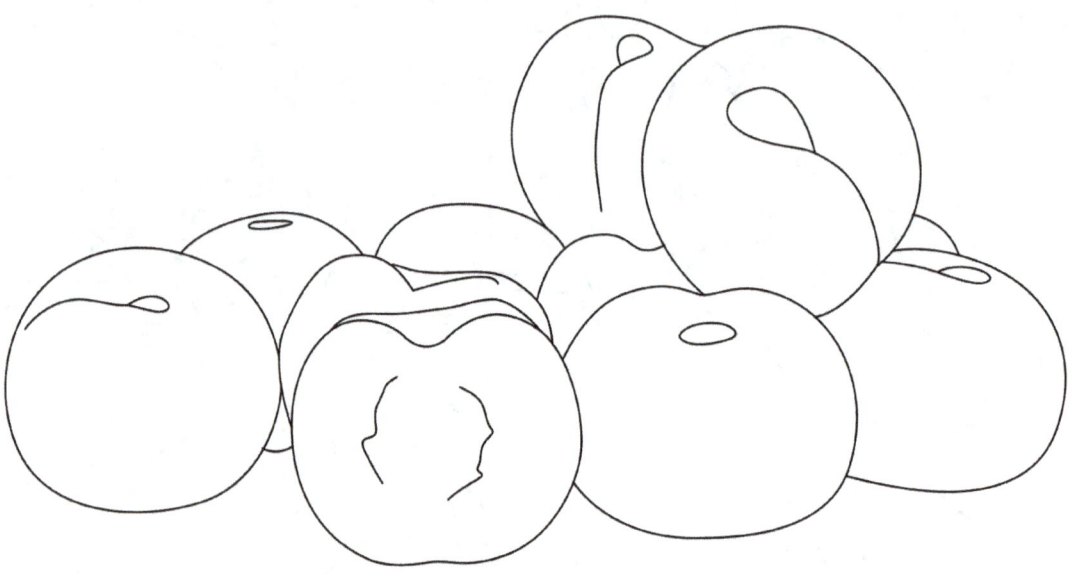

Plum
(pluhm)

relieves stomach pain, protects bone health, and prevents heart disease

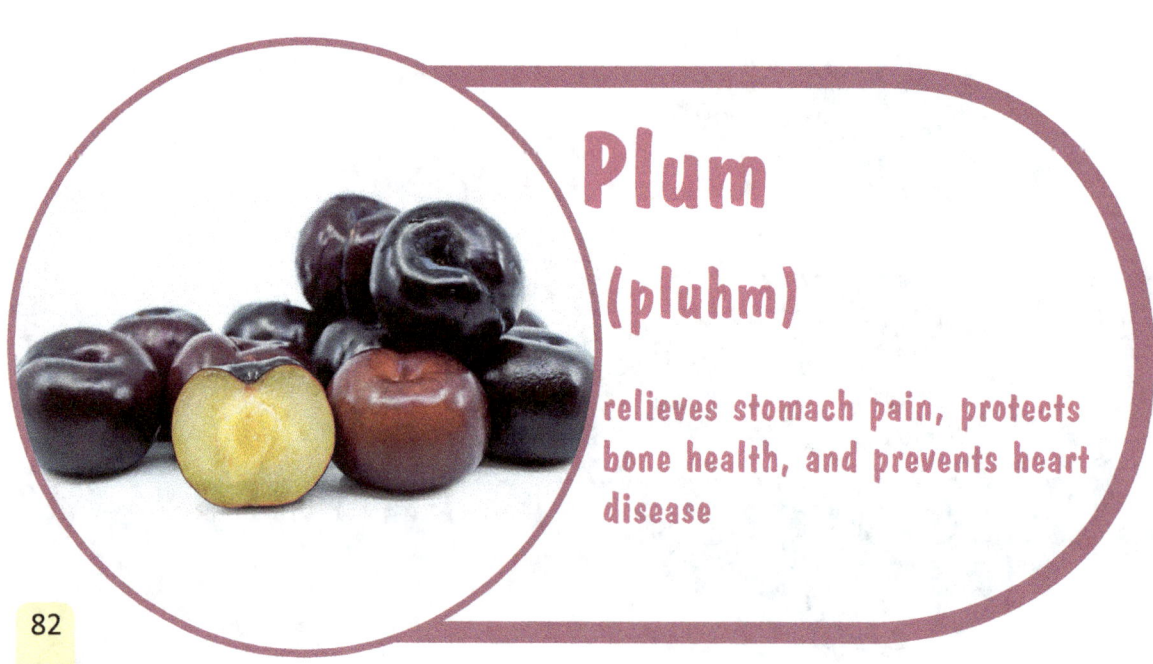

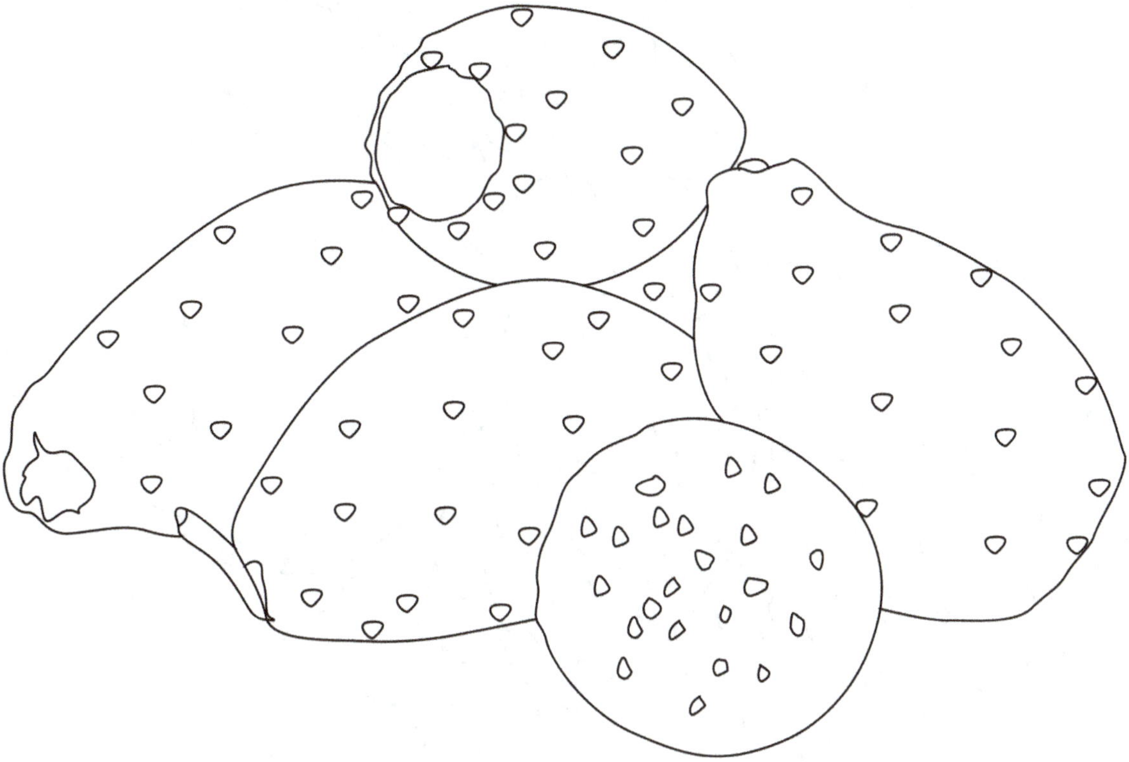

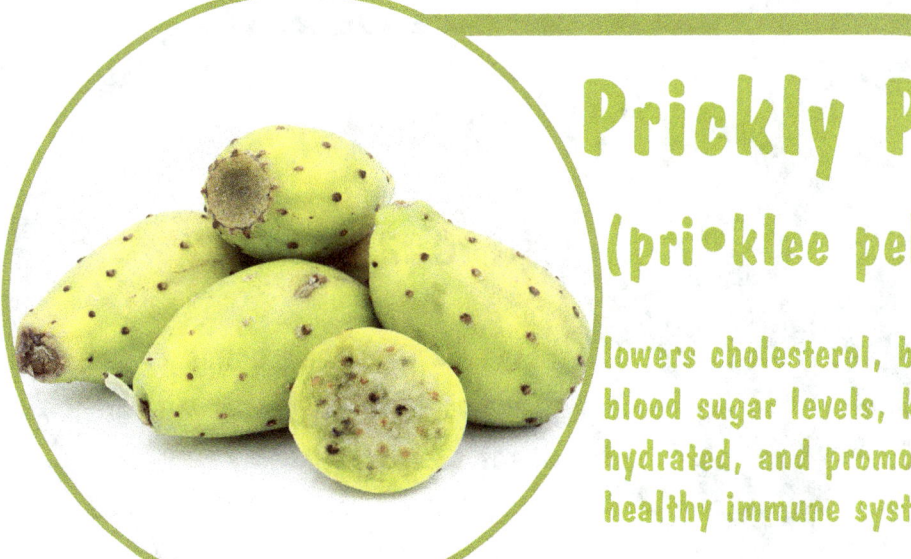

Prickly Pear
(pri•klee pehr)

lowers cholesterol, balances blood sugar levels, keeps skin hydrated, and promotes a healthy immune system

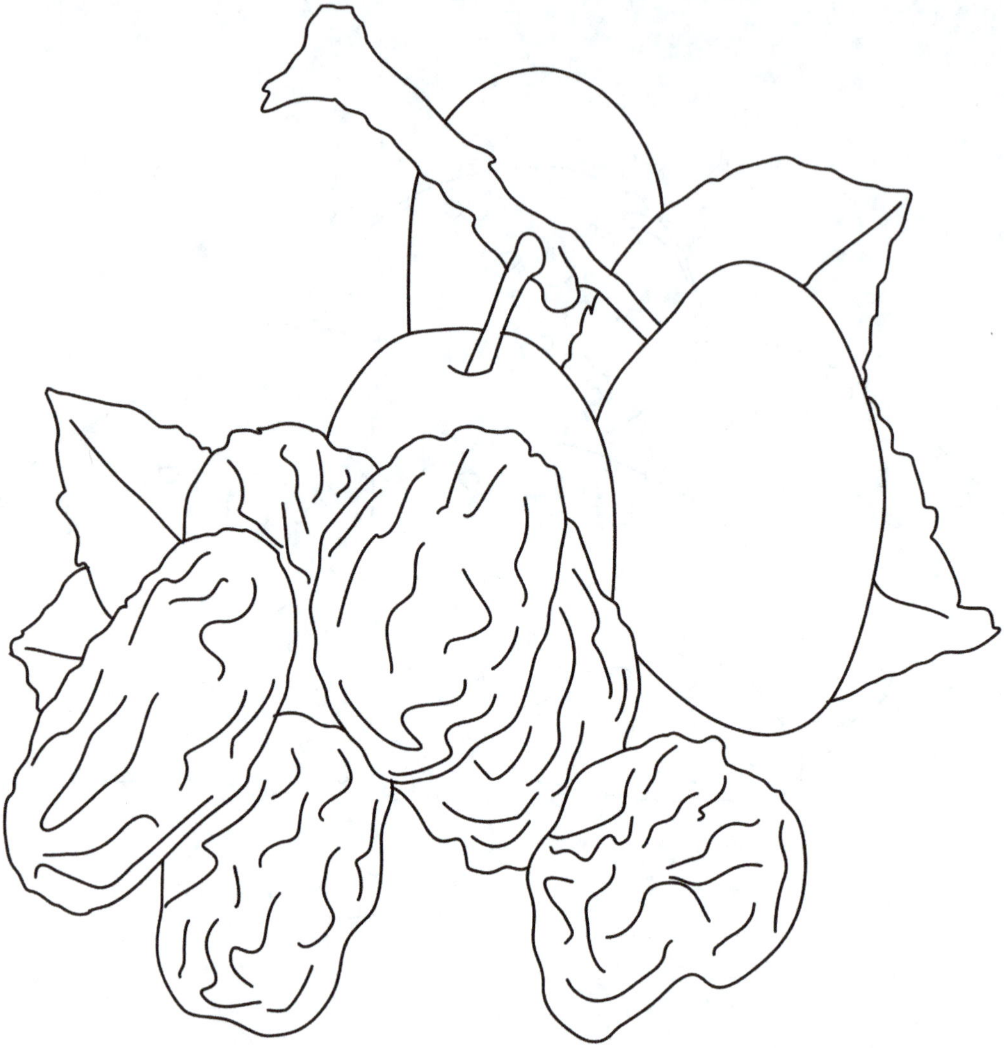

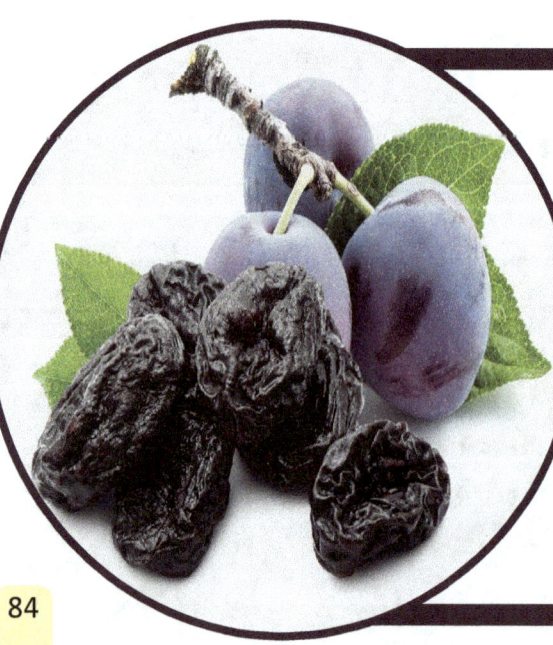

Prunes
(proonz)

helps build strong bones and muscles, and helps prevent an upset stomach

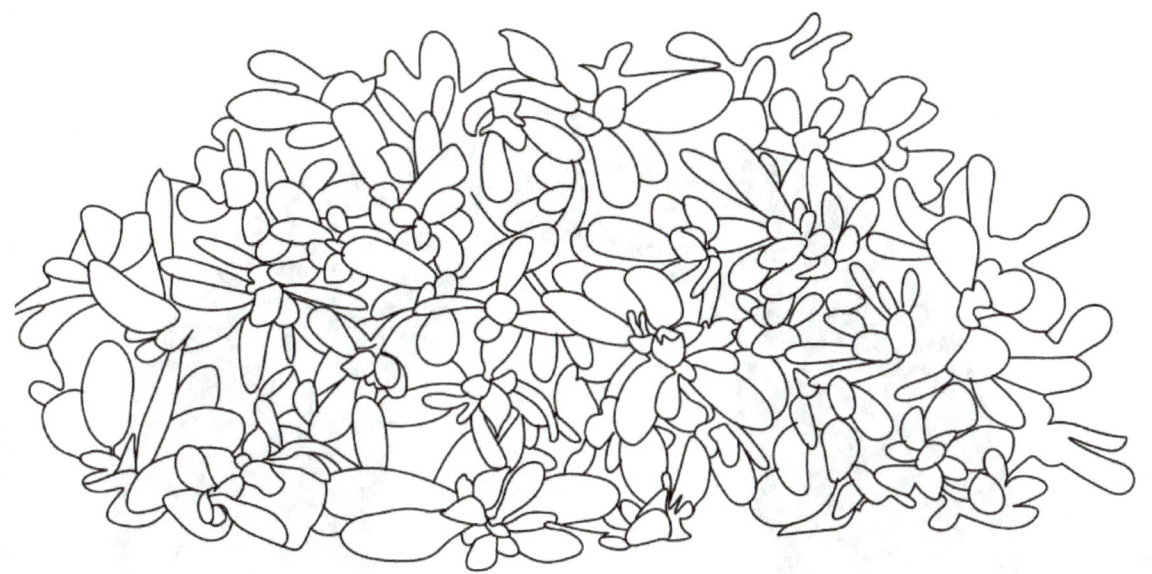

Purslane
(pur•sluhn)

source of healthy fatty acids, helps clean the blood, protects the lungs, and helps digestive tract

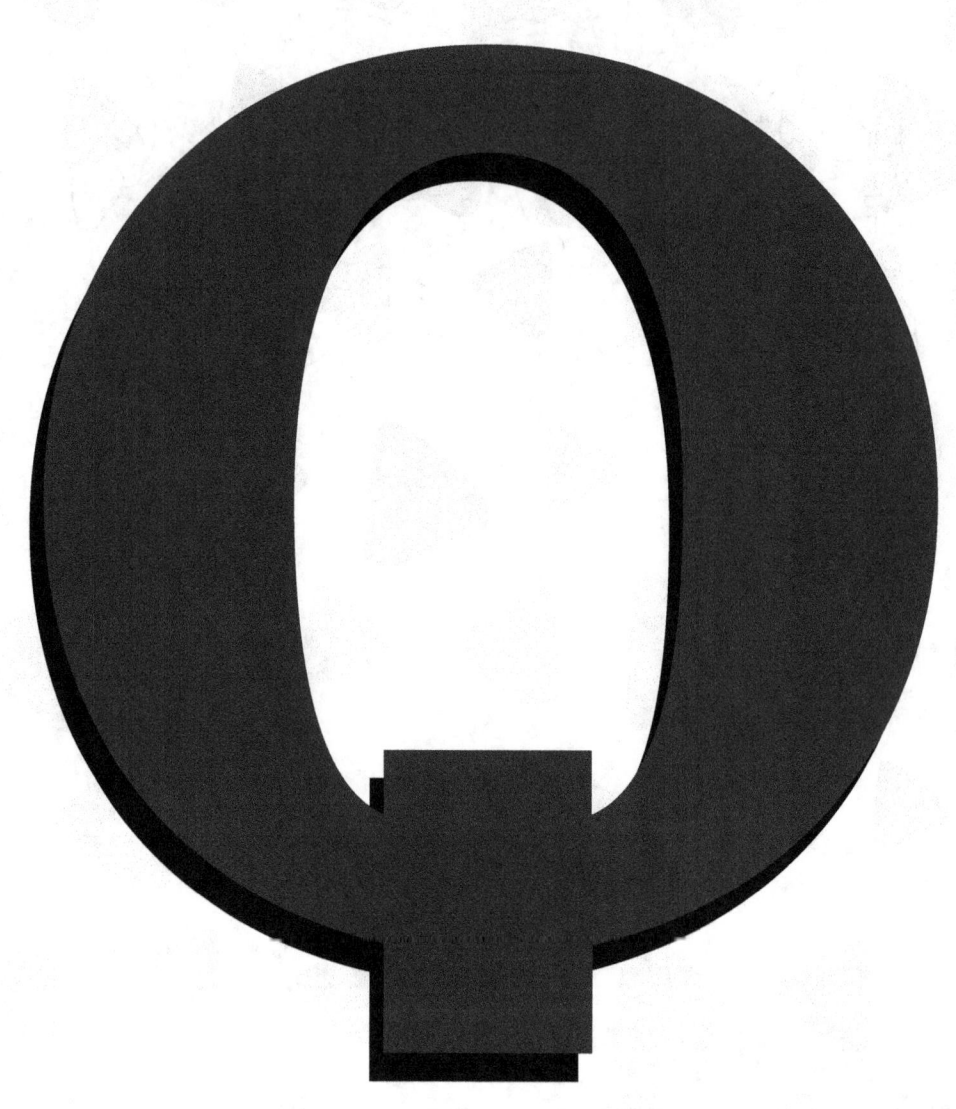

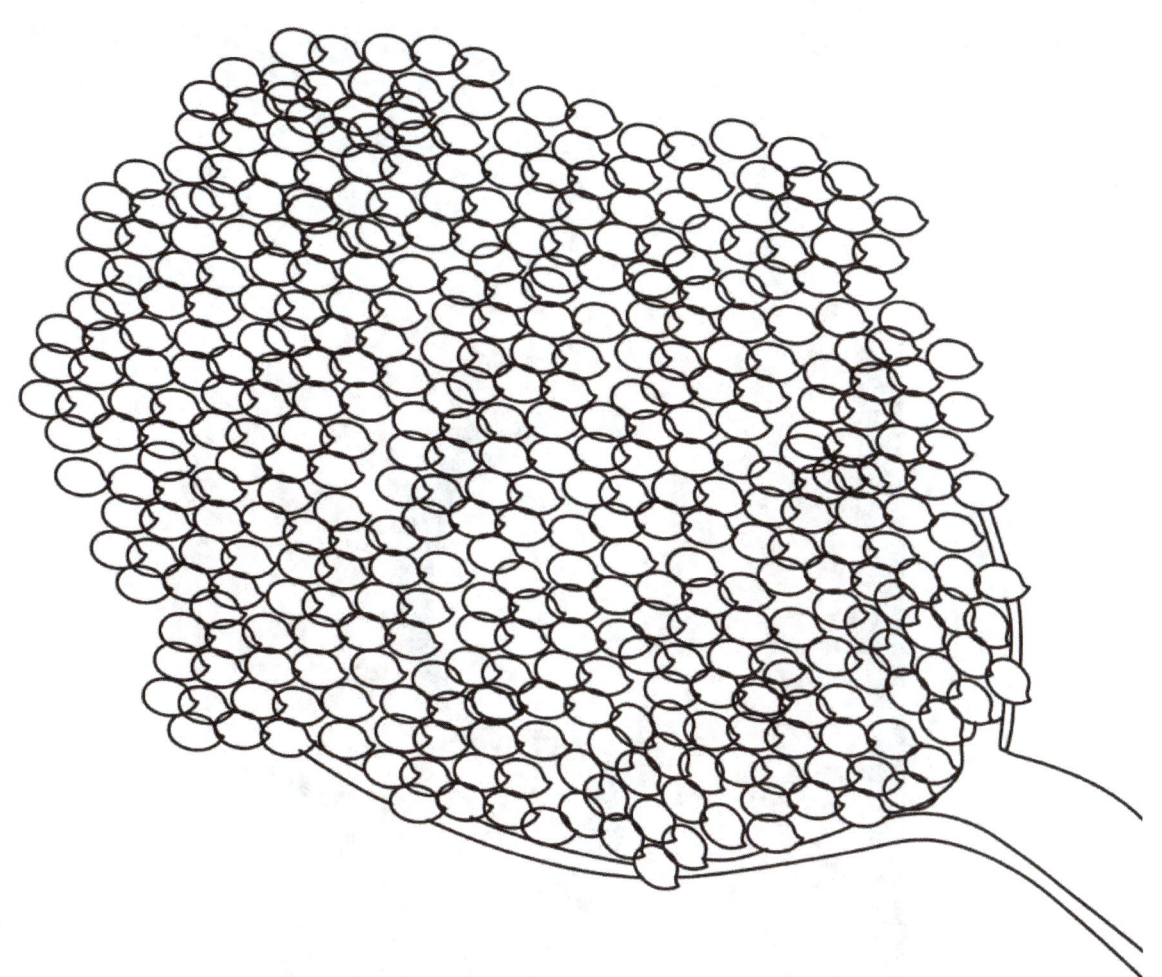

Quinoa
(keen•waa)

good source of amino acids and healthy fats, high in fiber, and promotes healthy muscle development

R

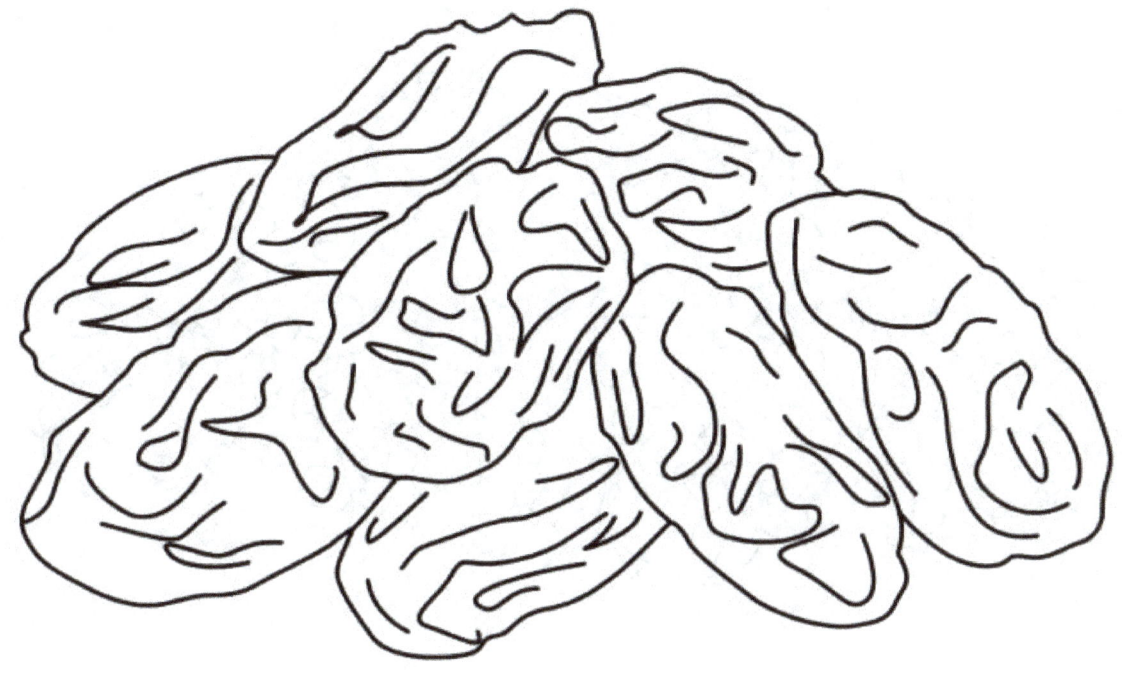

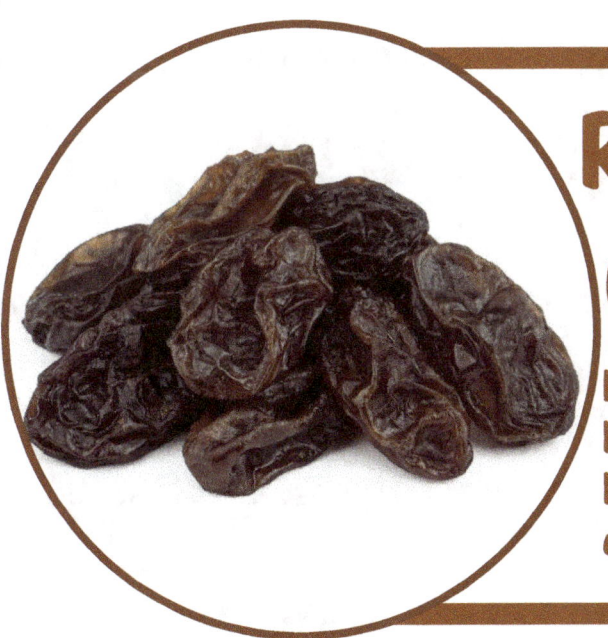

Raisin
(rei•zn)

lower risk of heart disease, helps reduce fevers, supports heart health, and protects the eyes and teeth

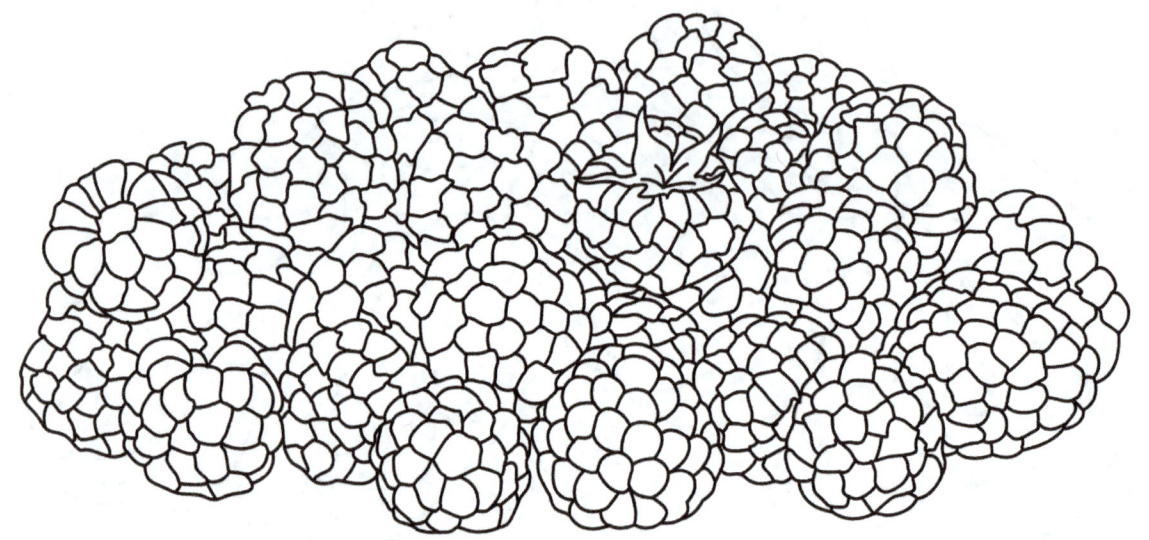

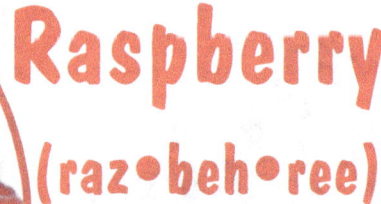

Raspberry
(raz•beh•ree)

promotes heart function, good source of fatty acids, and helps prevent cardiovascular diseases

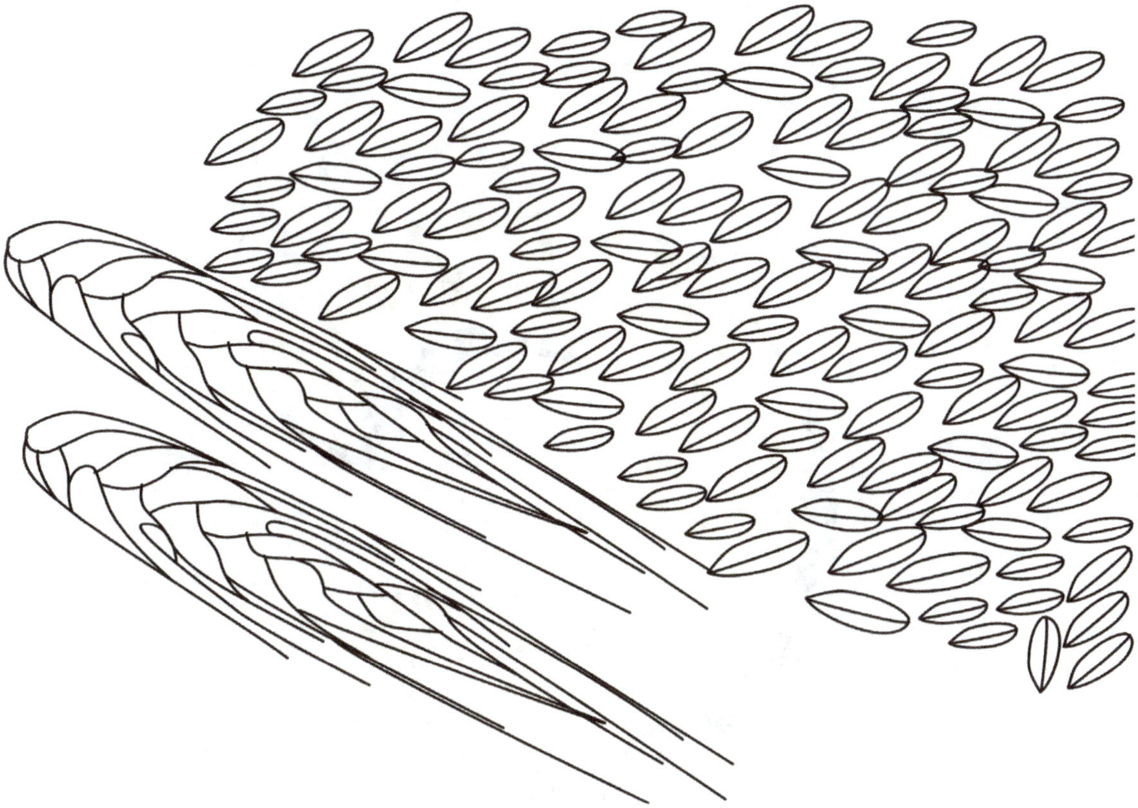

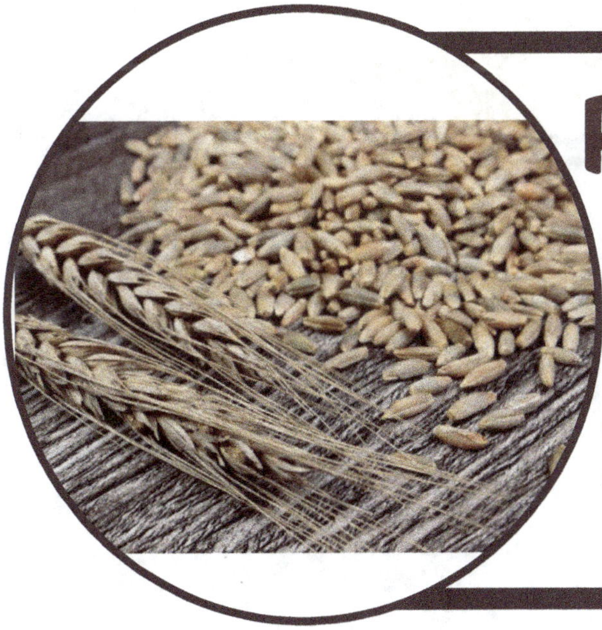

Rye
(rai)

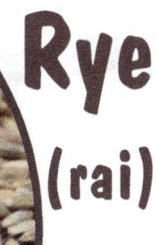

reduce risks of cancer and blood disease, lowers cholesterol, and supports healthy muscle growth

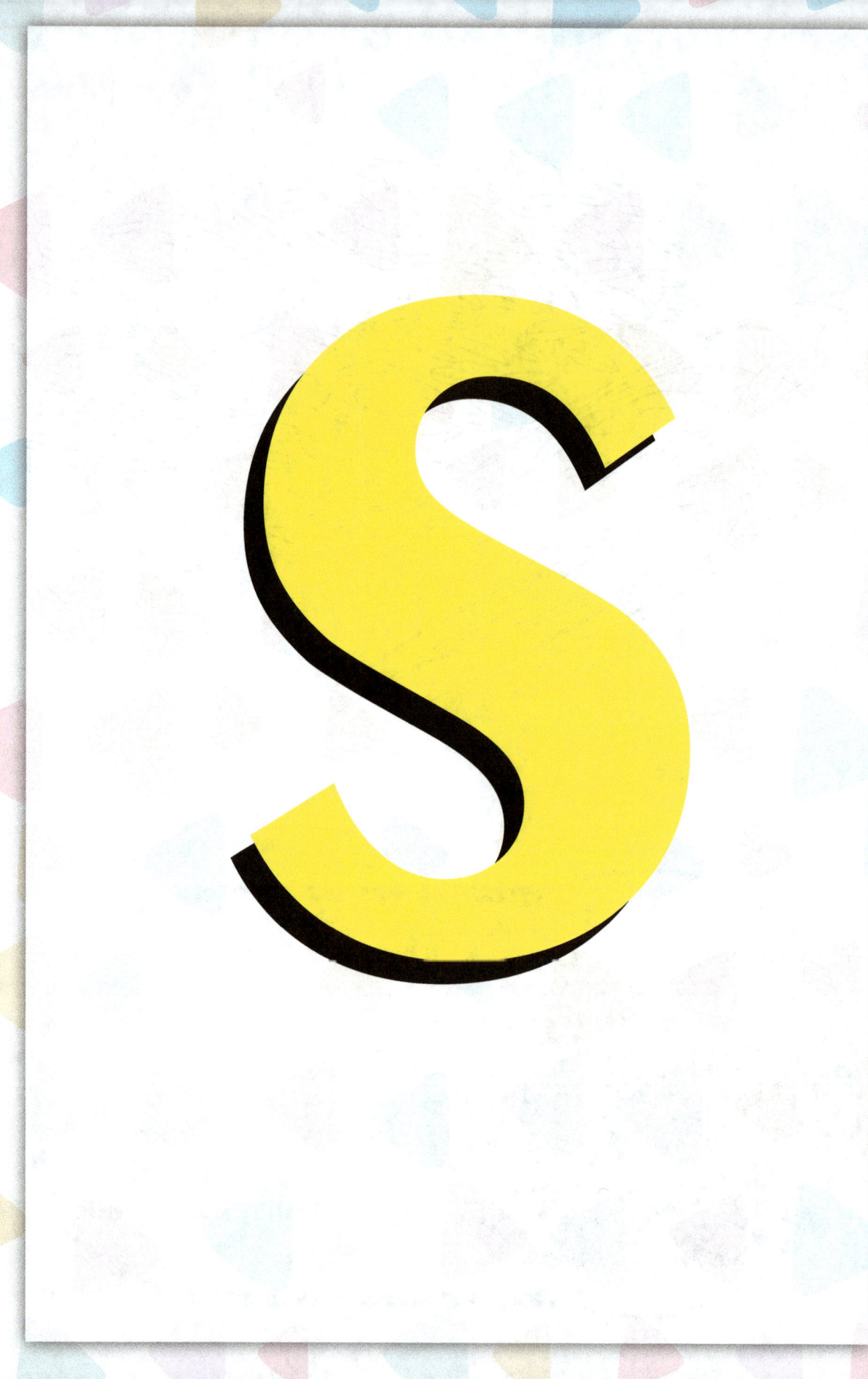

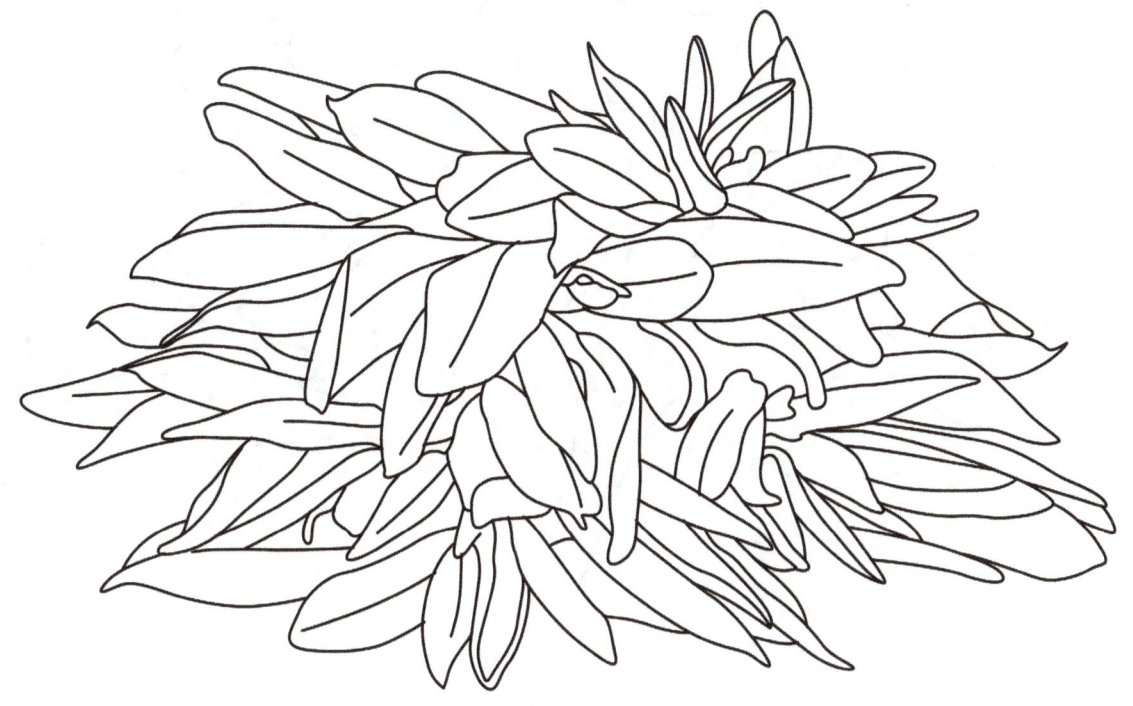

Sage
(seij)

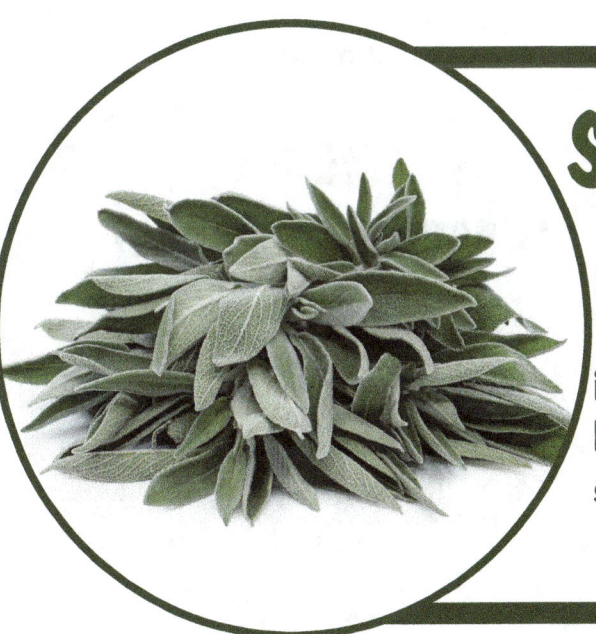

improve memory and brain health, relieve headaches and sore throat, and improves mood

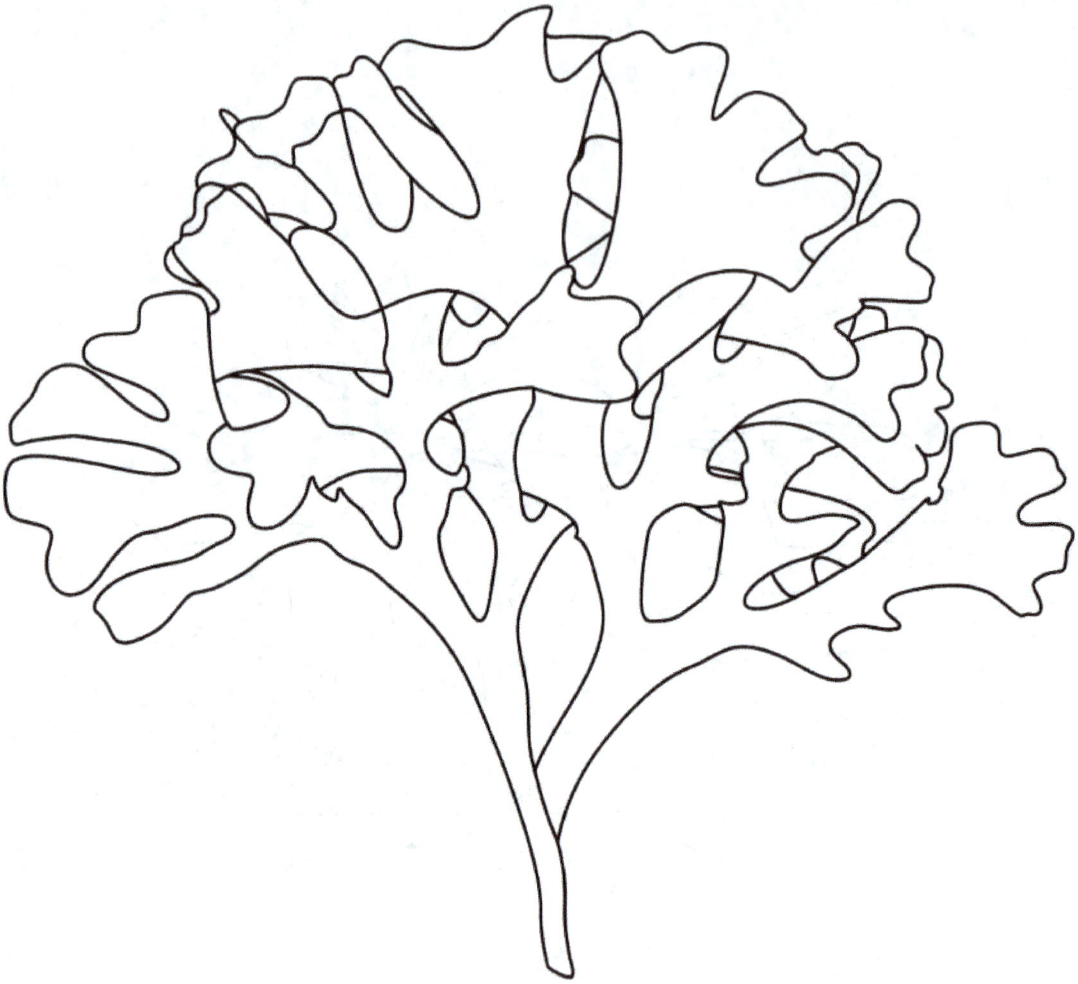

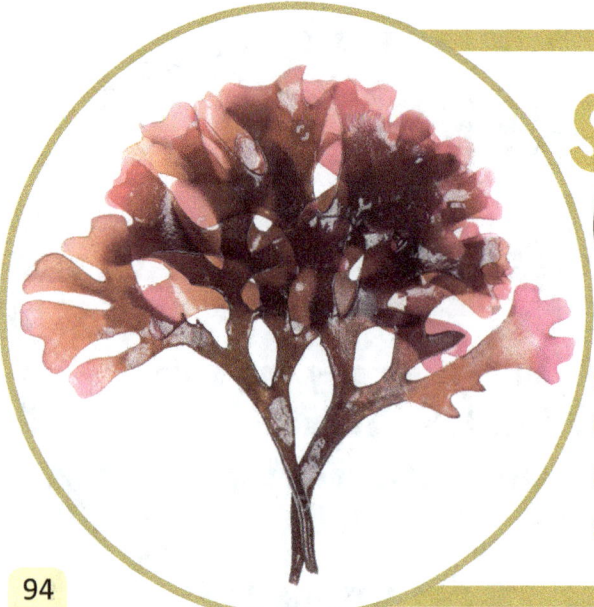

Sea Moss
(Chondrus Crispus)
(see maas)

great source of calcium and essential minerals, helps remove mucus in the body, and promotes skin, hair, and nail health

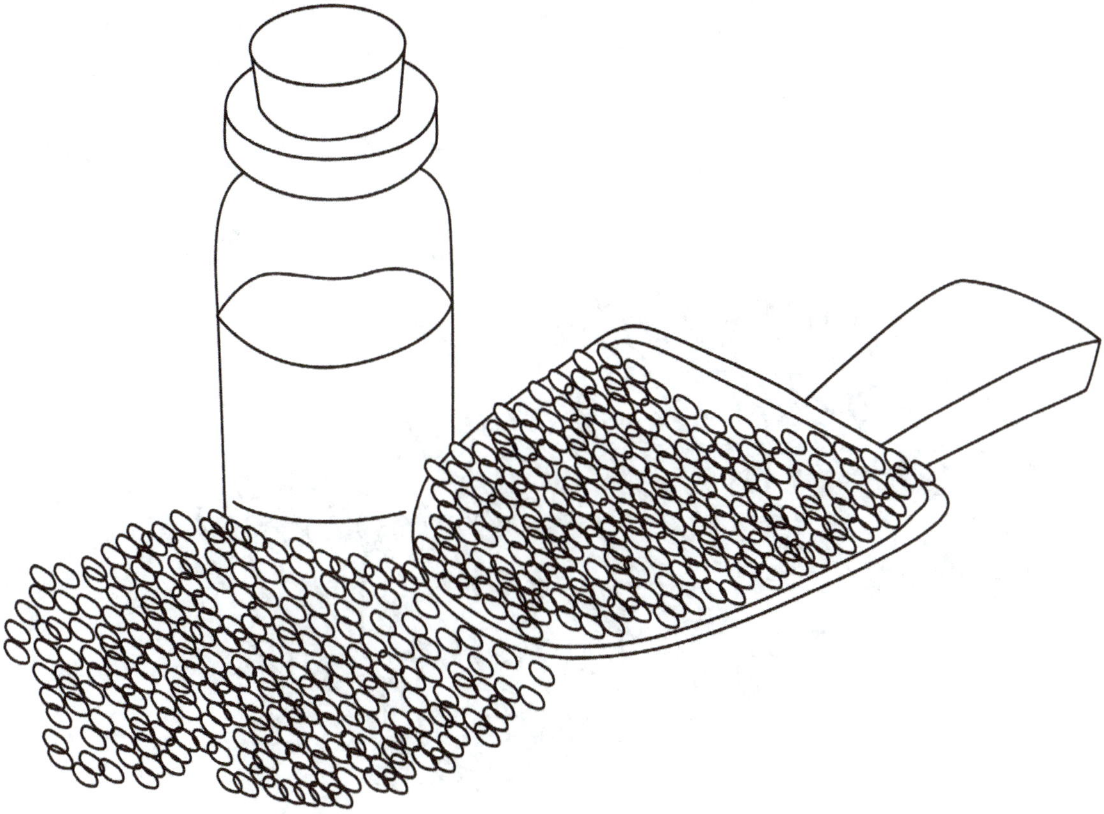

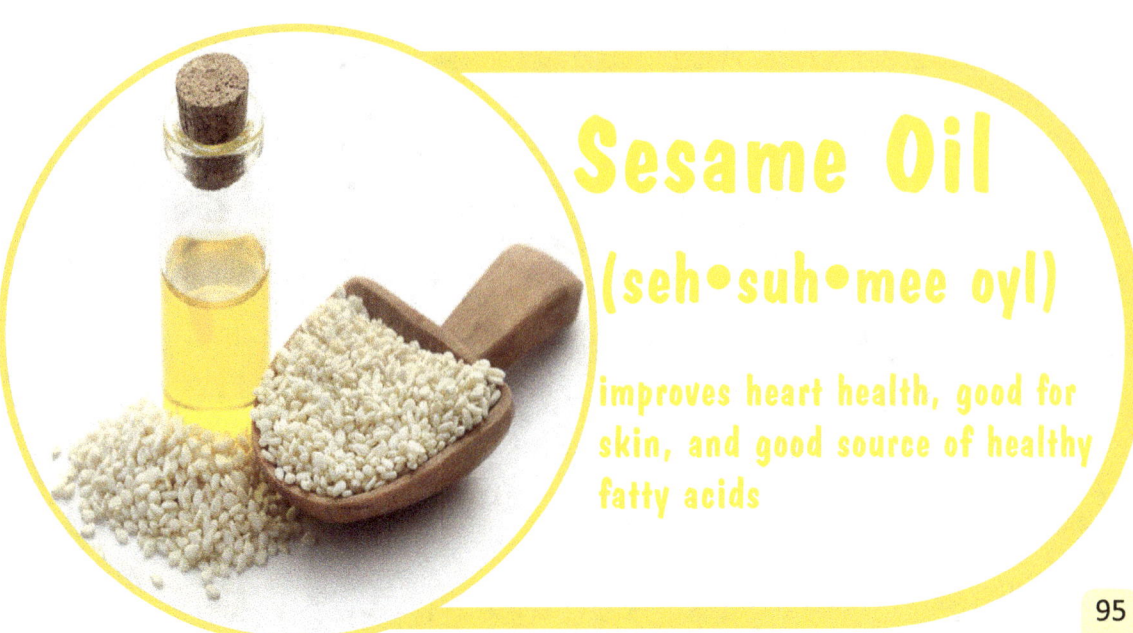

Sesame Oil
(seh•suh•mee oyl)

improves heart health, good for skin, and good source of healthy fatty acids

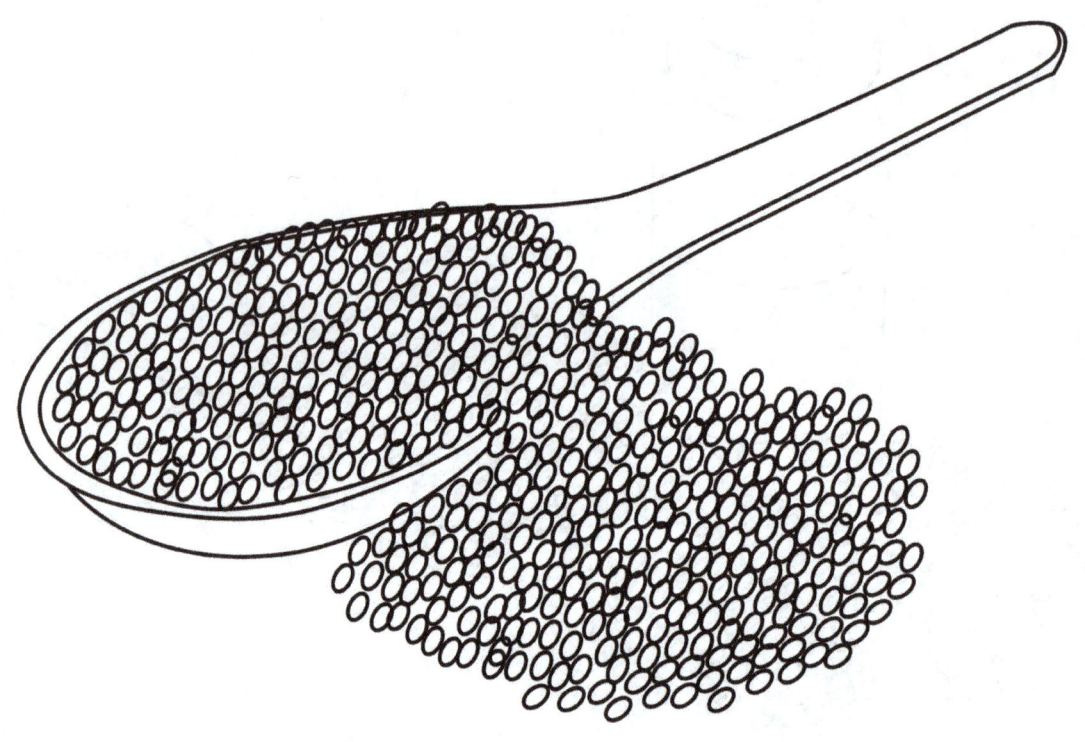

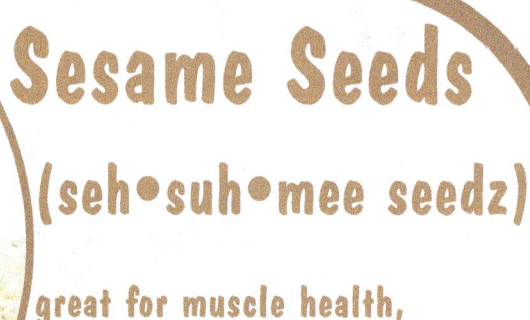

Sesame Seeds
(seh•suh•mee seedz)

great for muscle health, supports healthy bones, and contains healthy fats

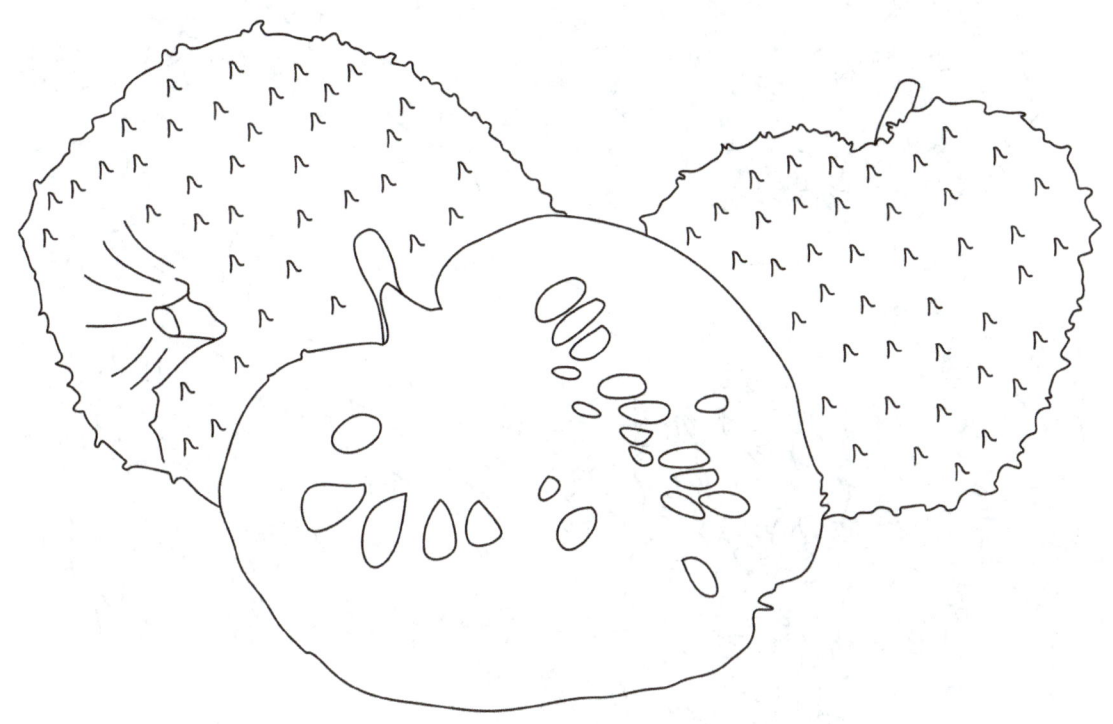

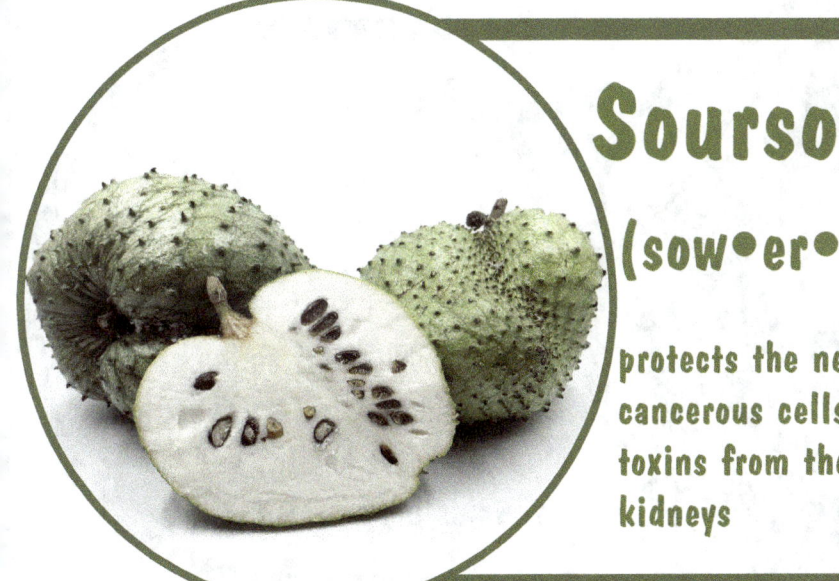

Soursop
(sow•er•saap)

protects the nerves, kills cancerous cells, and removes toxins from the blood and kidneys

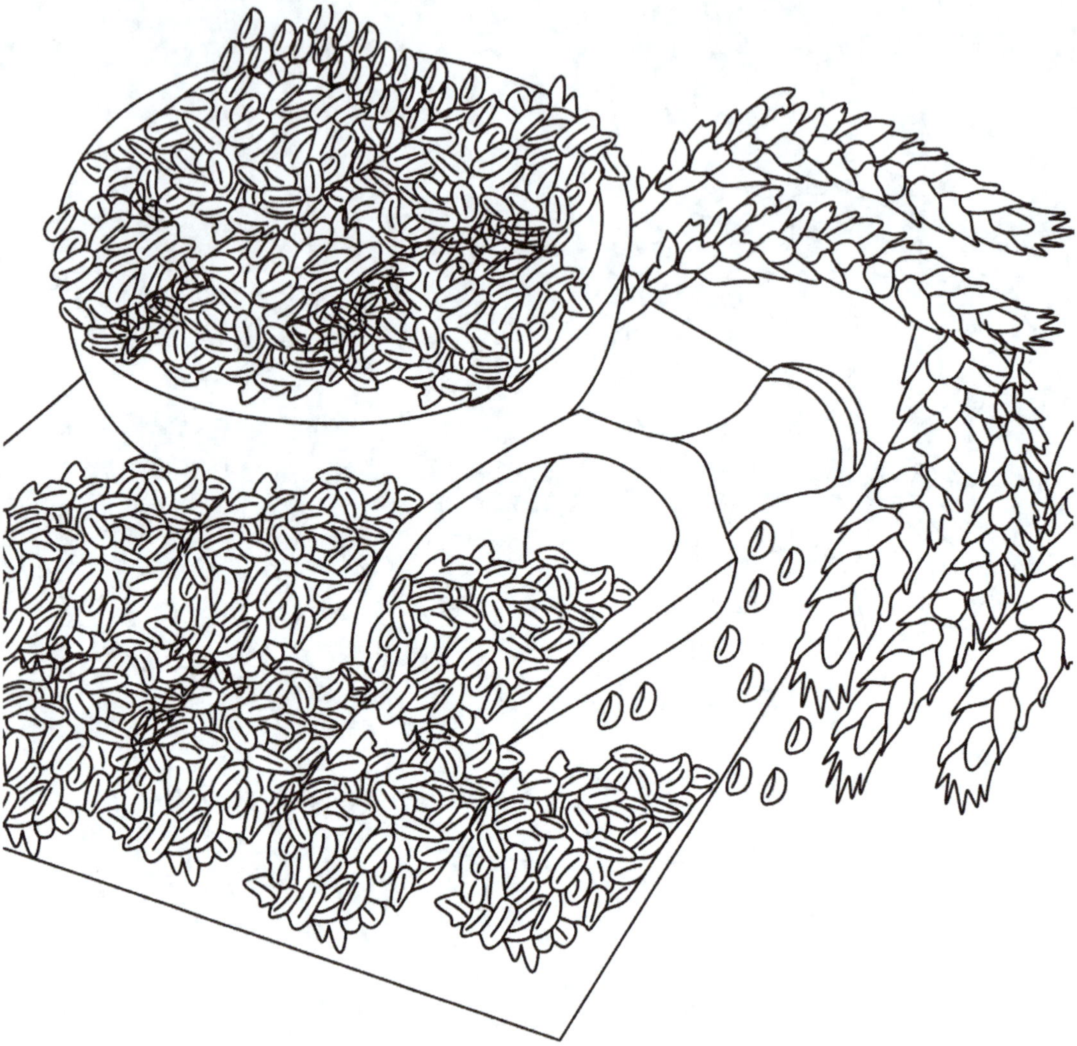

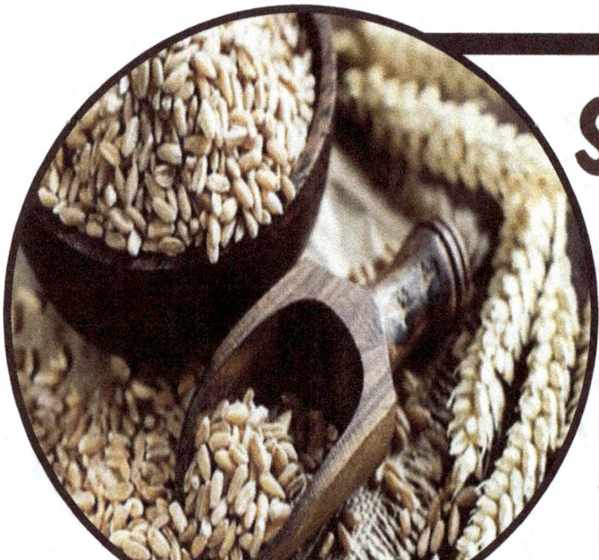

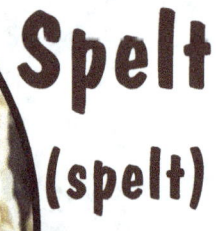

Spelt
(spelt)

important source of amino acids, healthy carbohydrates, and fiber, supports heart health, and maintains bone health

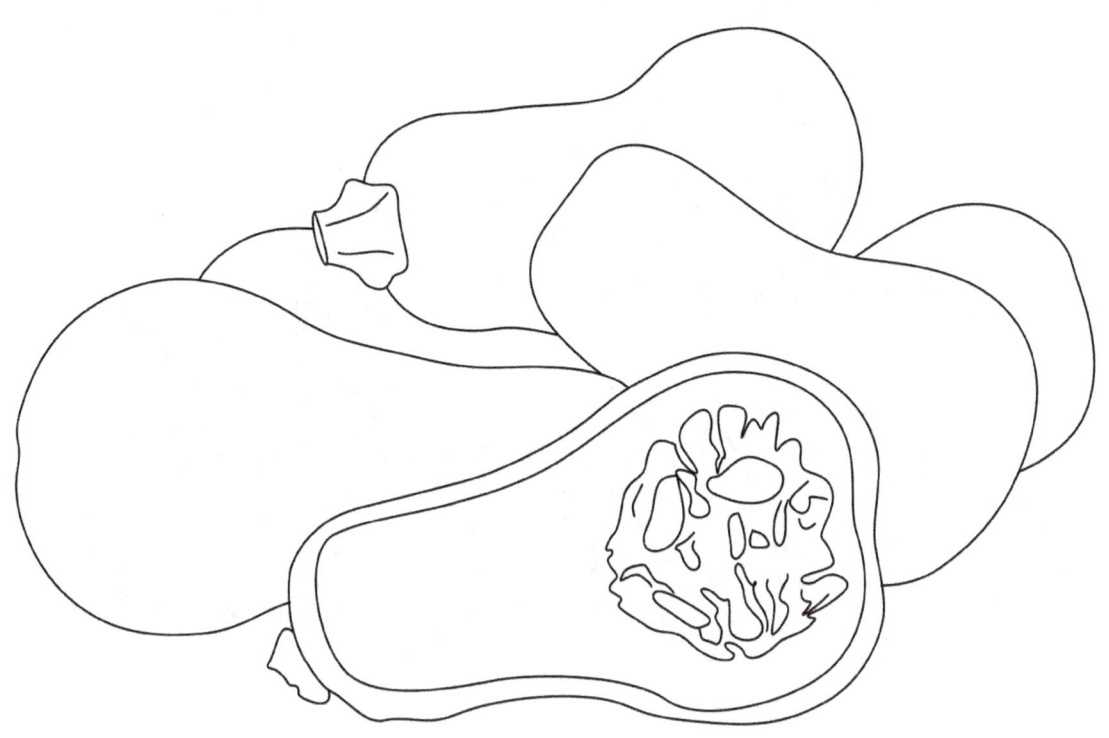

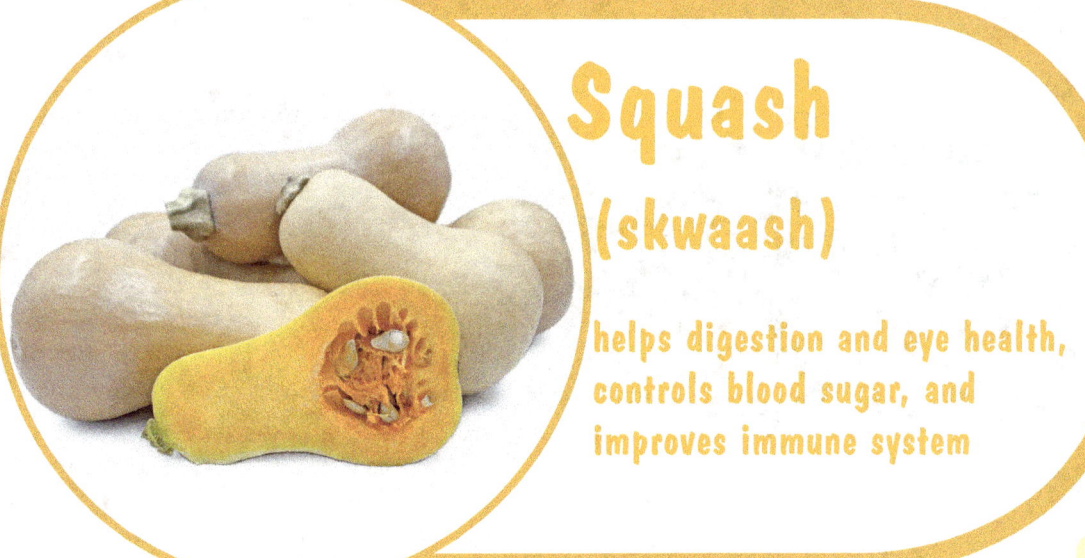

Squash
(skwaash)

helps digestion and eye health, controls blood sugar, and improves immune system

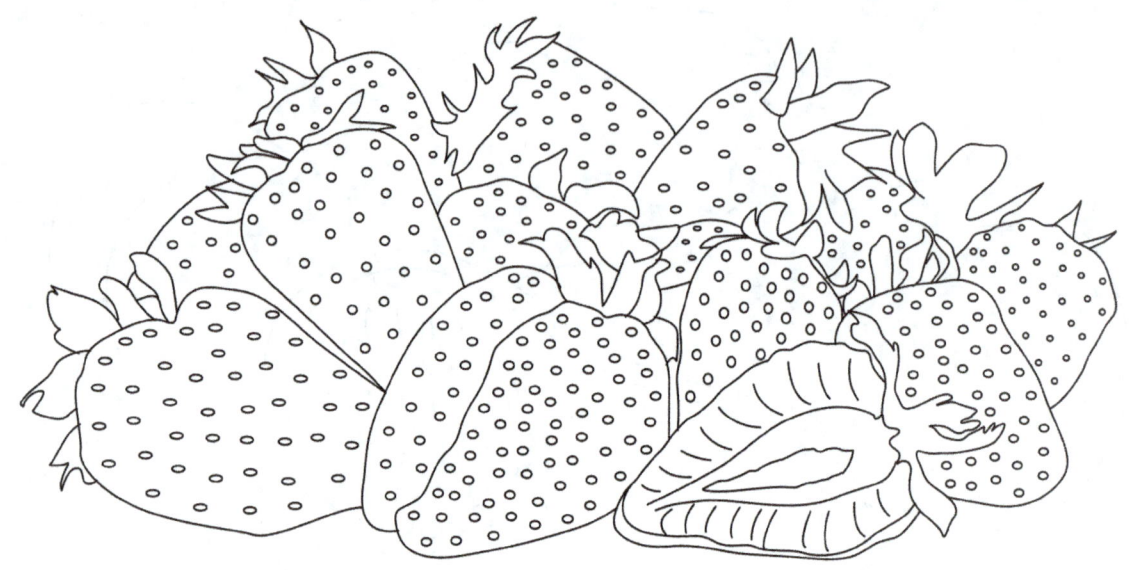

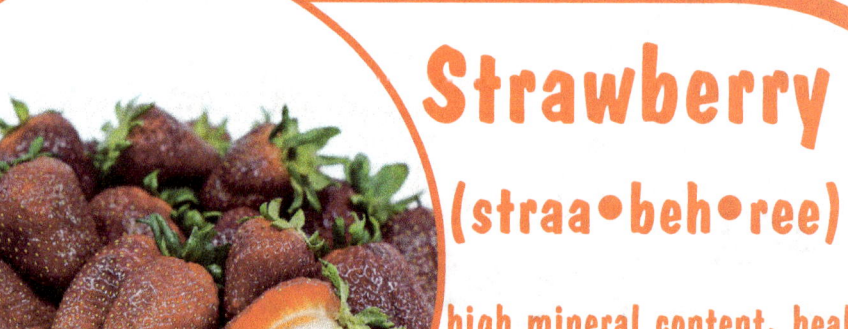

Strawberry
(straa•beh•ree)

high mineral content, healthy for skin, boosts immune system, and improves brain function

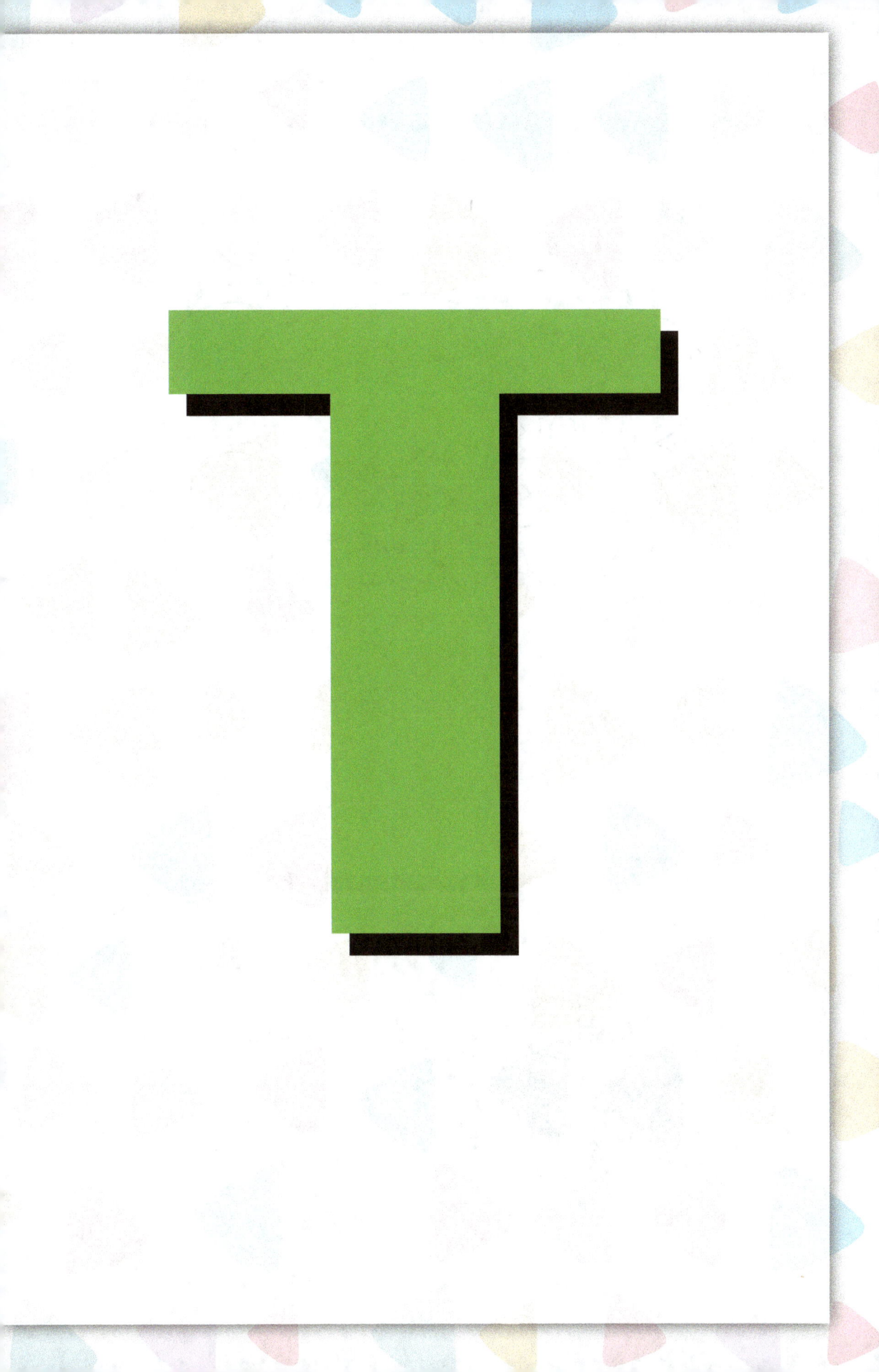

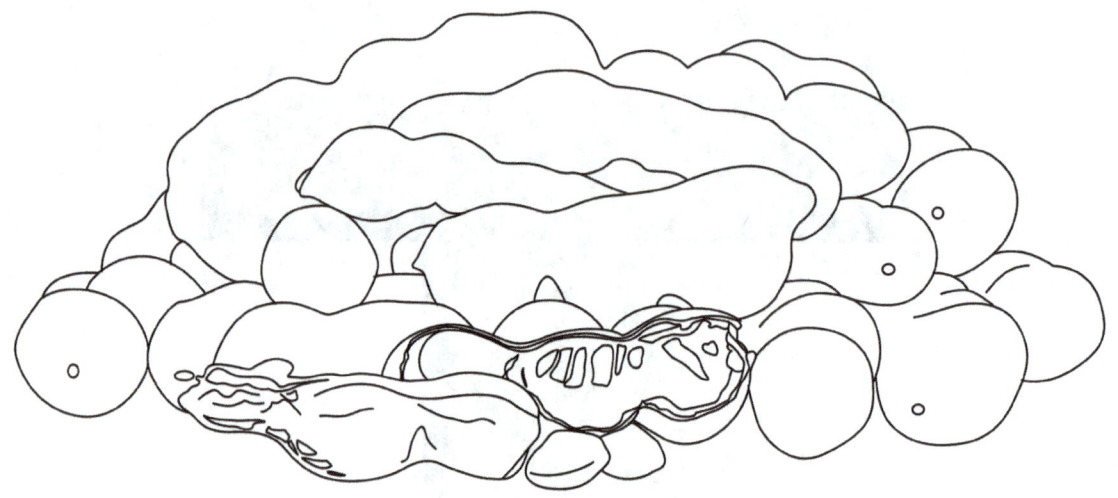

Tamarind
(ta•mr•uhnd)

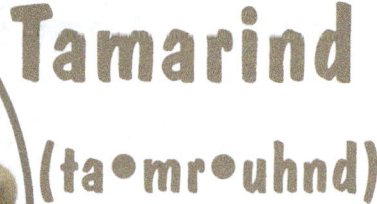

protects against cancer, lowers blood sugar, and helps stimulate digestion

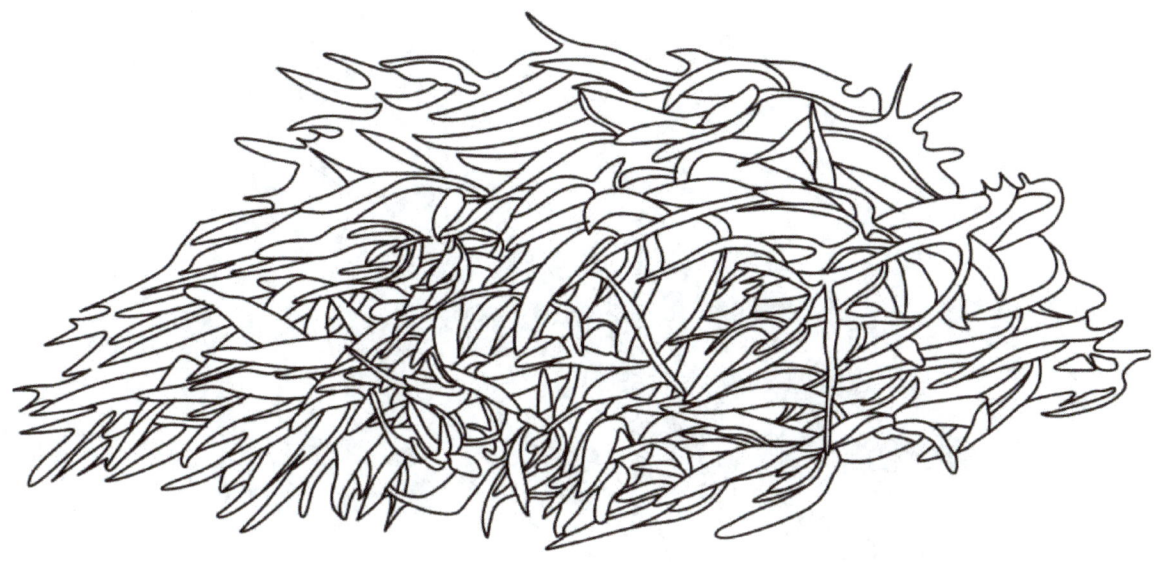

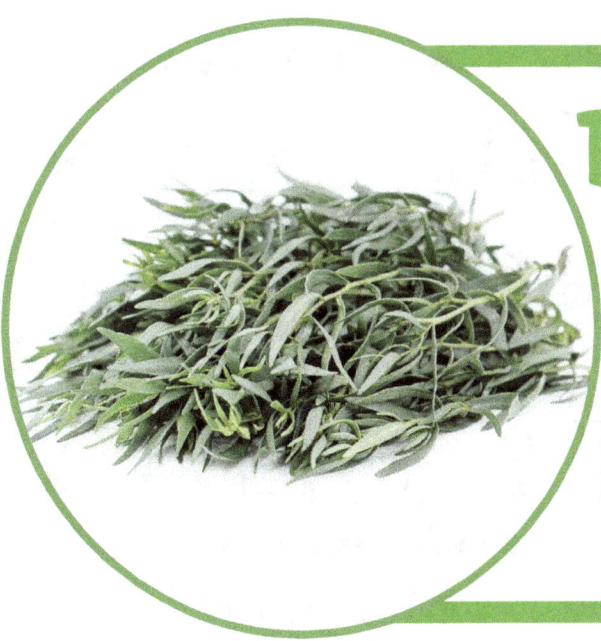

Tarragon
(teh•ruh•gaan)

improves sleep, helps with digestion, improves appetite, and prevents stomach pain

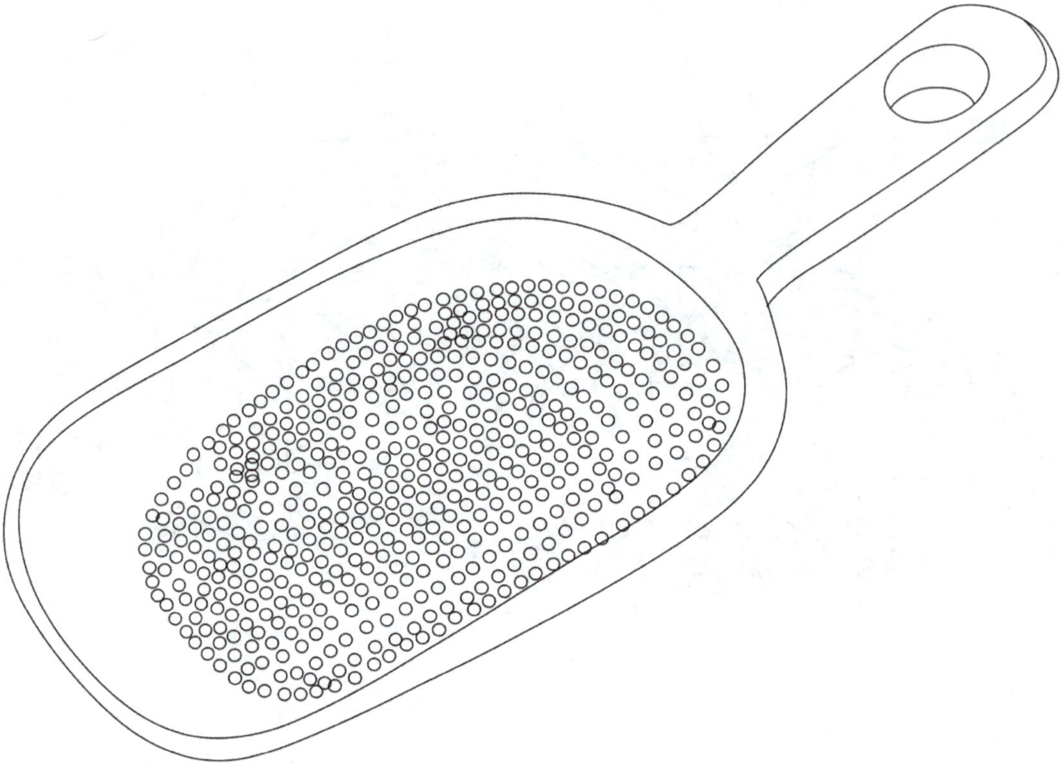

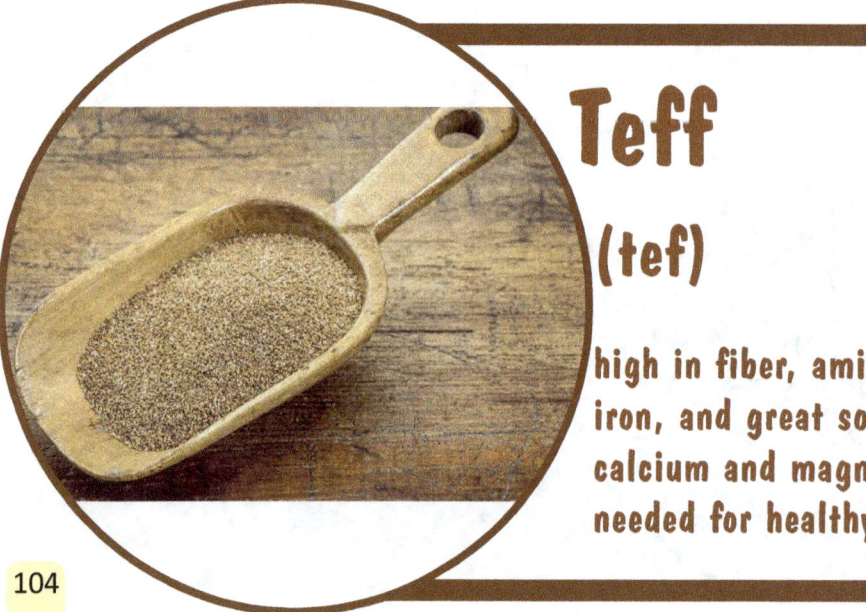

Teff
(tef)

high in fiber, amino acids, and iron, and great source of calcium and magnesium needed for healthy bones

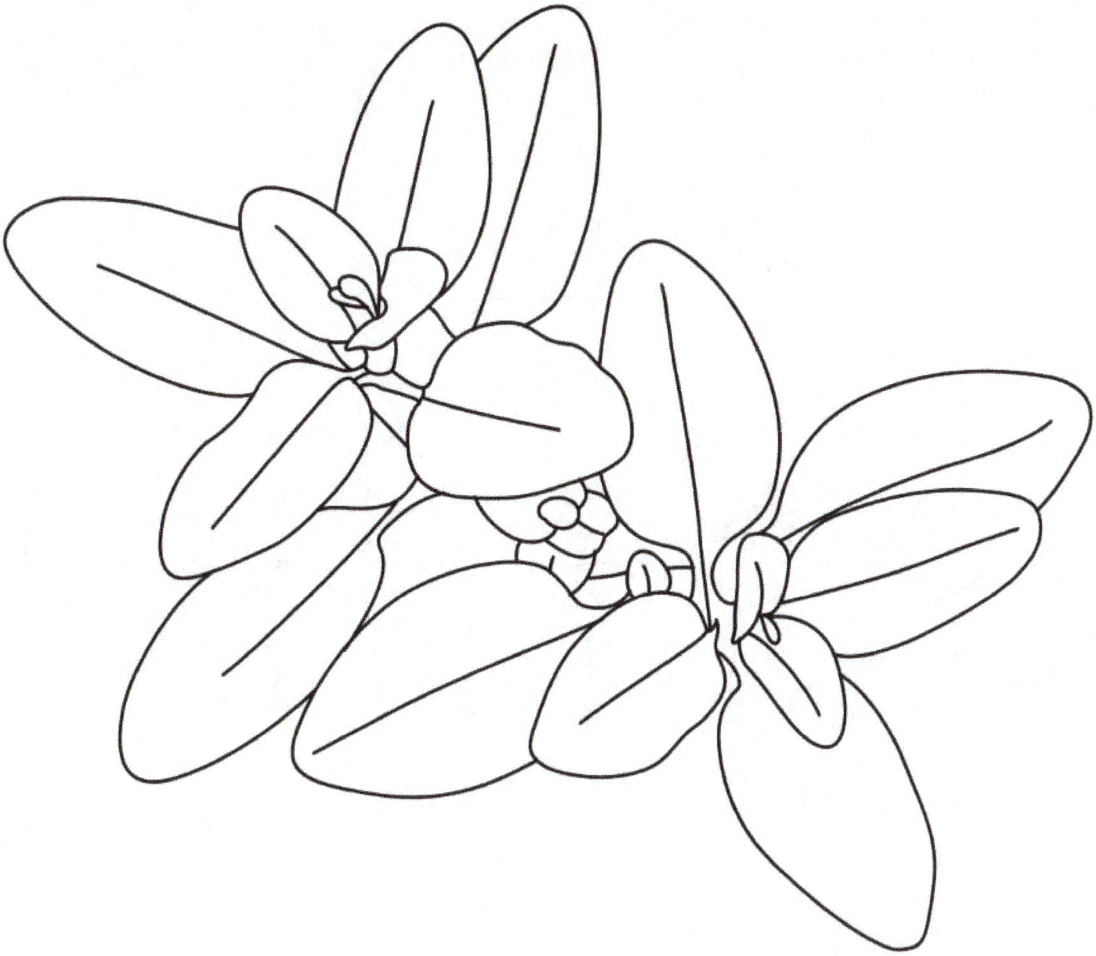

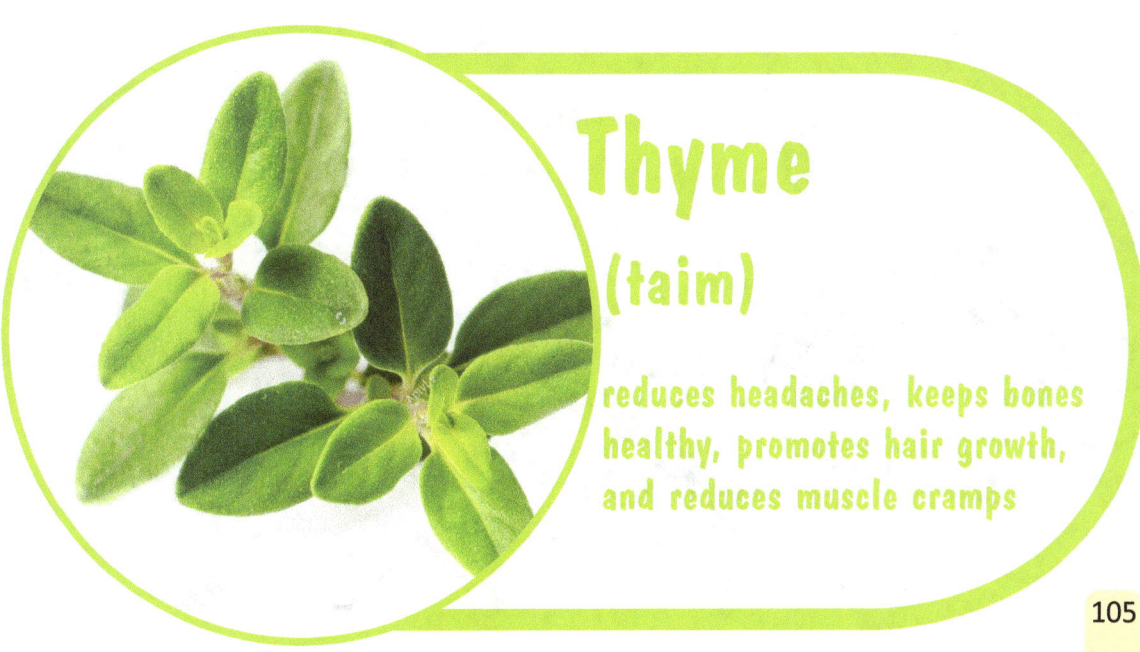

Thyme
(taim)

reduces headaches, keeps bones healthy, promotes hair growth, and reduces muscle cramps

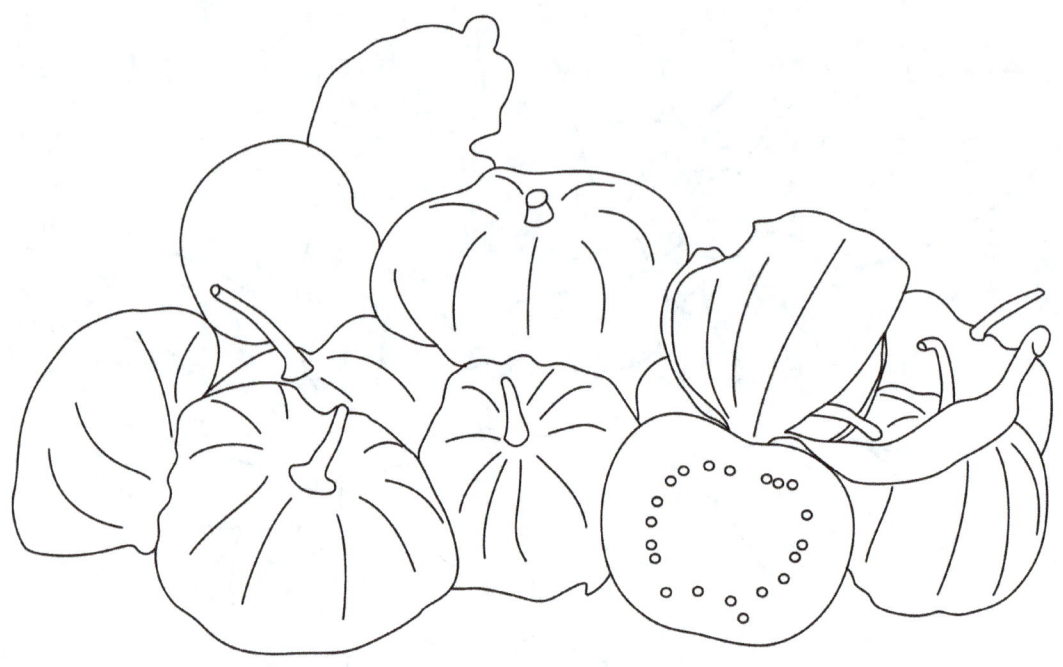

Tomatillo
(tow•muh•tee•ow)

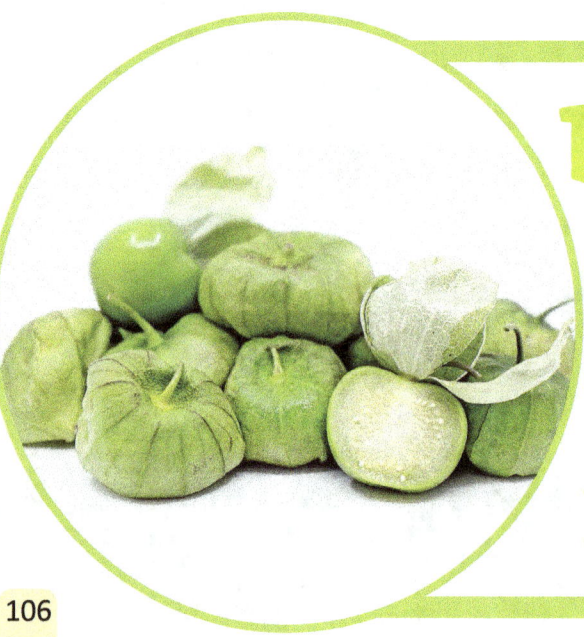

boosts immune system, reduce inflammation, improves energy, and protects the skin and eye cells

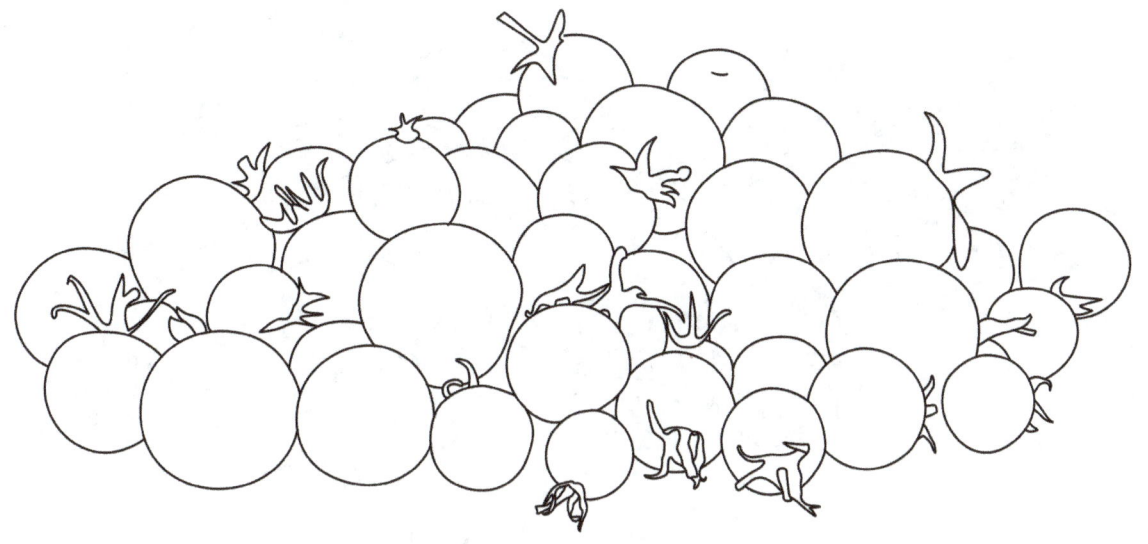

Tomato
(tuh•mei•tow)

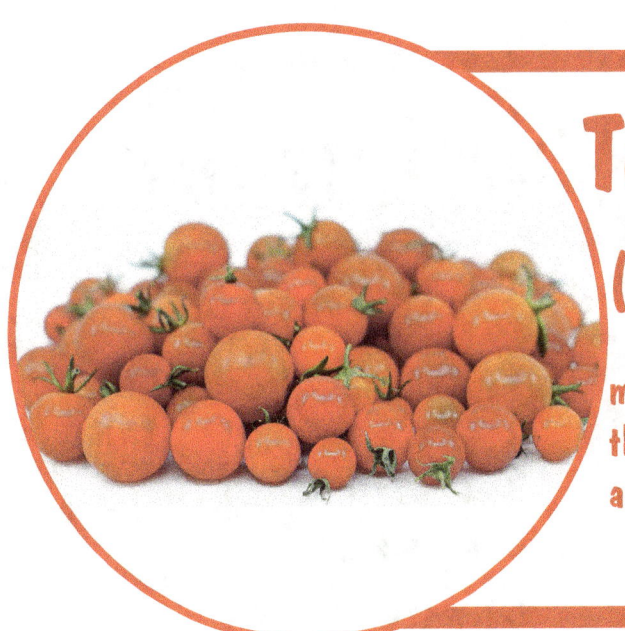

maintains hydration, protects the cells, promotes heart health, and fights against cancer

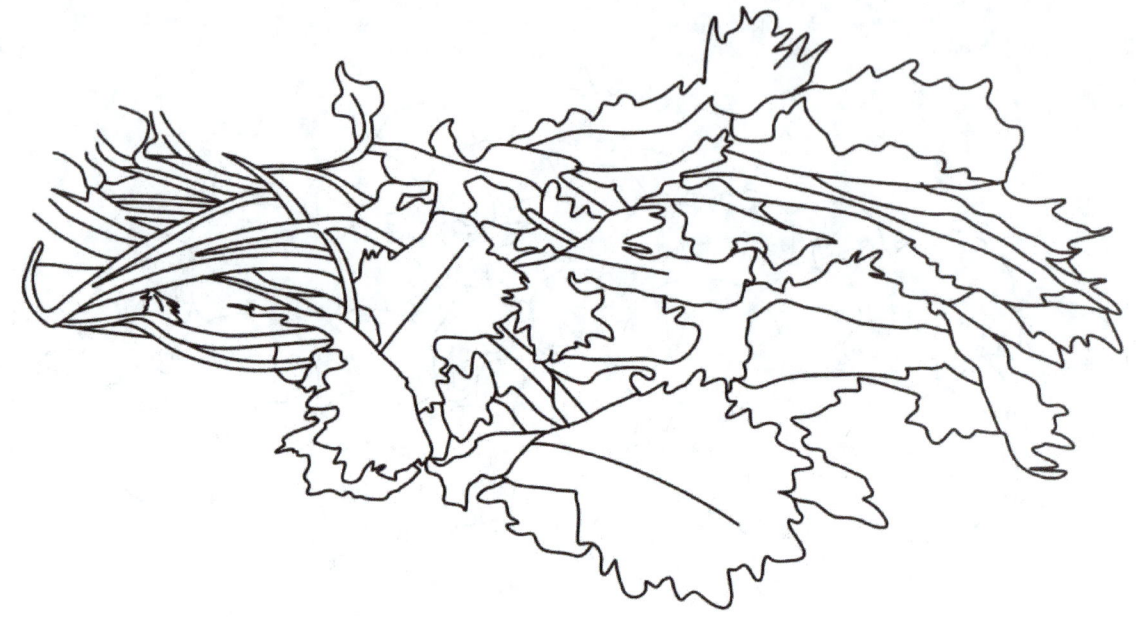

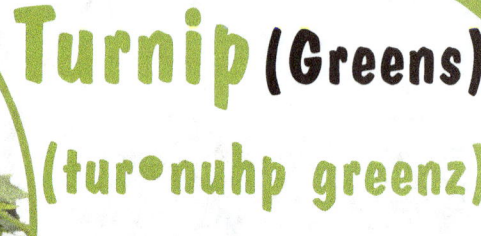

Turnip (Greens)
(tur•nuhp greenz)

keeps the skin and hair healthy, improves liver function, and fights against diseases like diabetes, heart disease and cancer

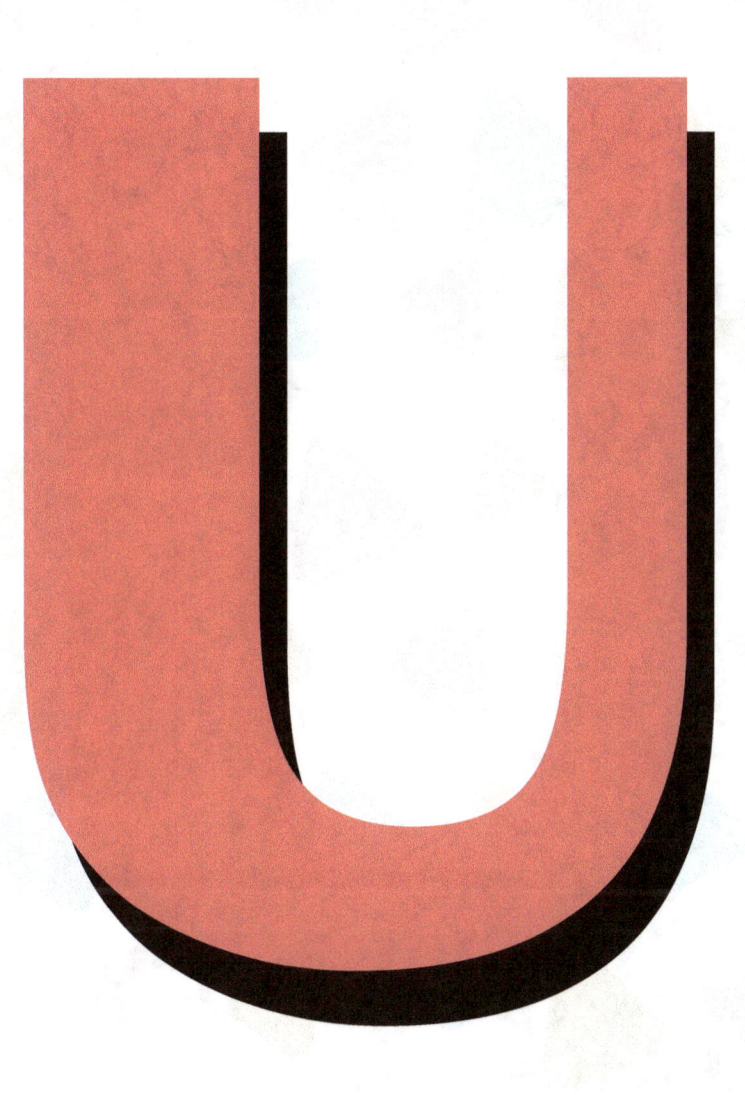

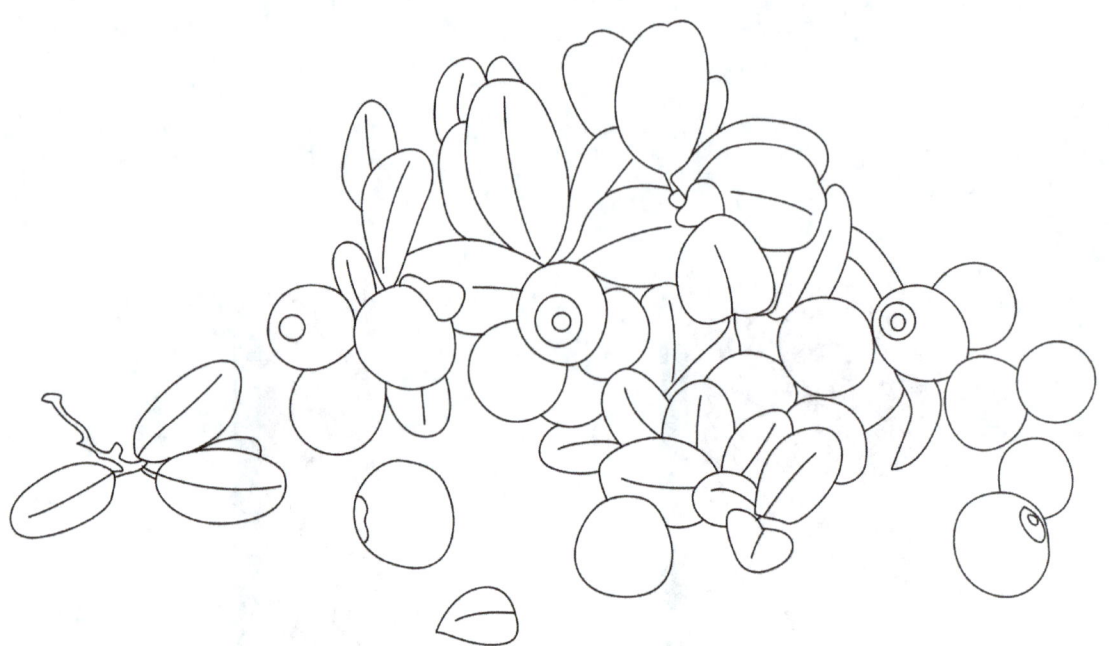

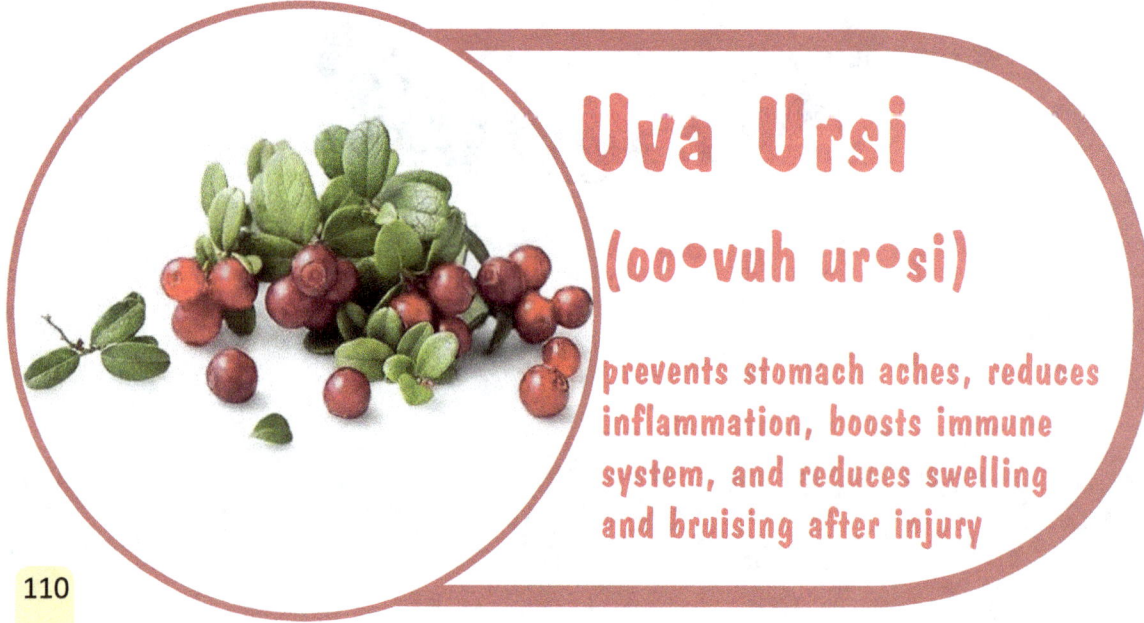

Uva Ursi
(oo•vuh ur•si)

prevents stomach aches, reduces inflammation, boosts immune system, and reduces swelling and bruising after injury

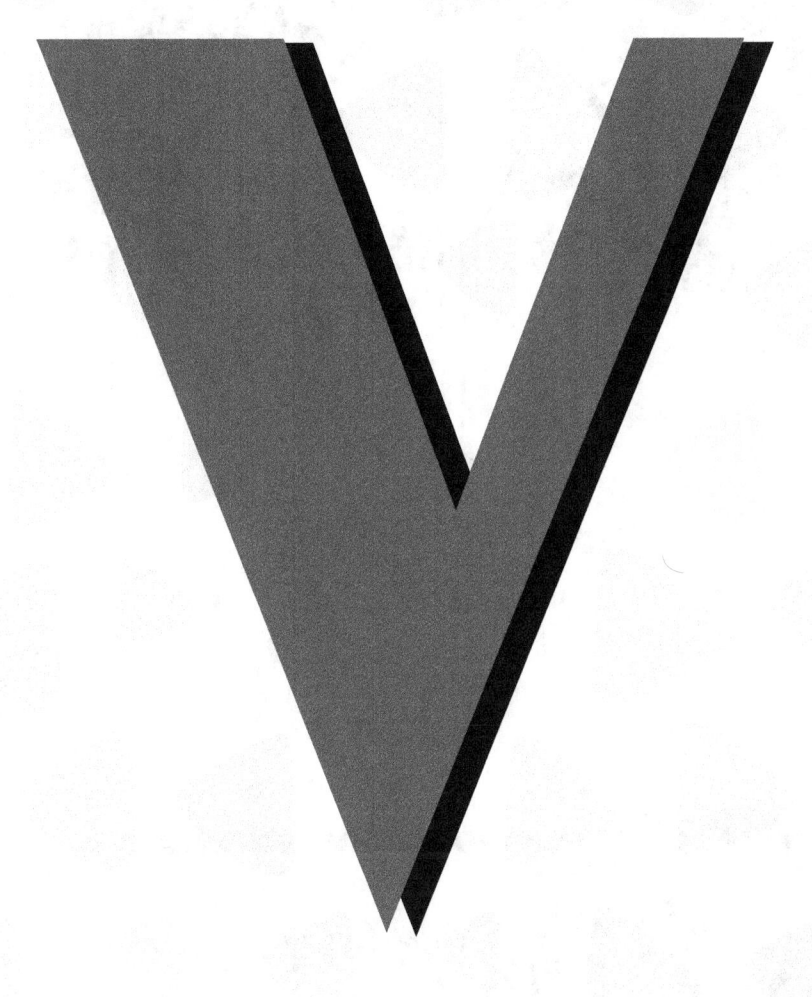

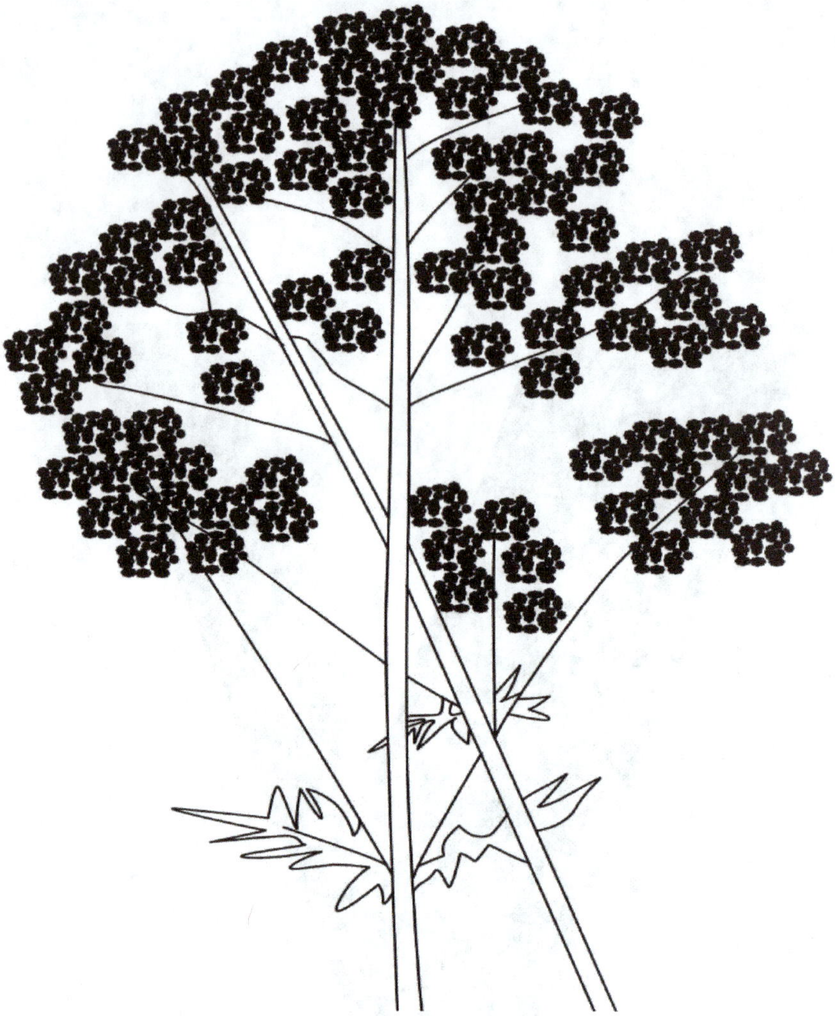

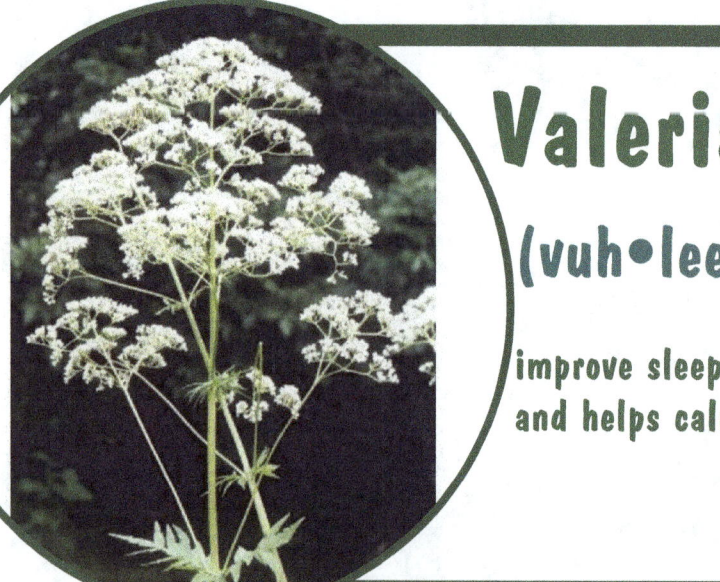

Valerian
(vuh•lee•ree•uhn)

improve sleep, relaxes nerves, and helps calm the body

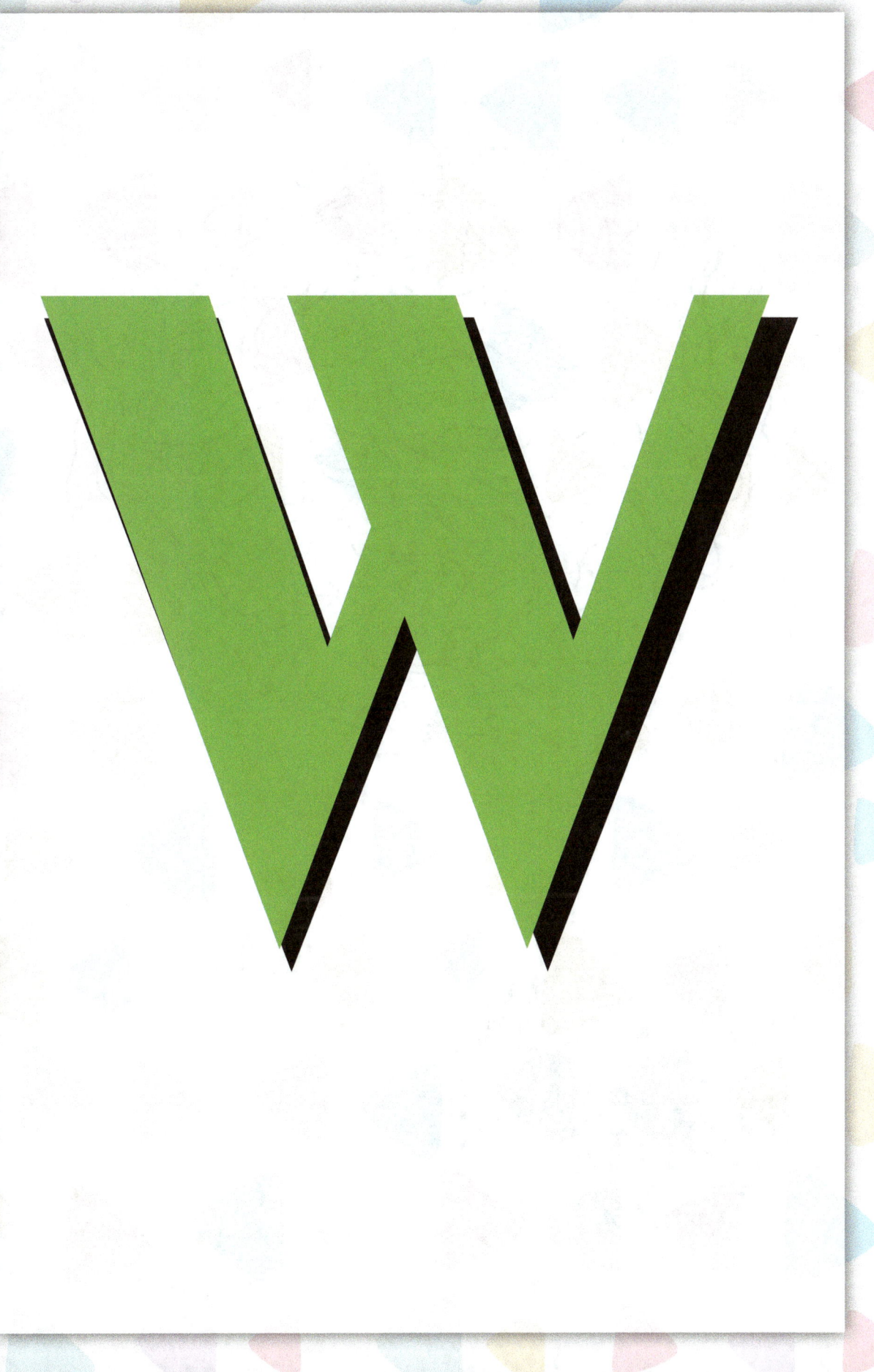

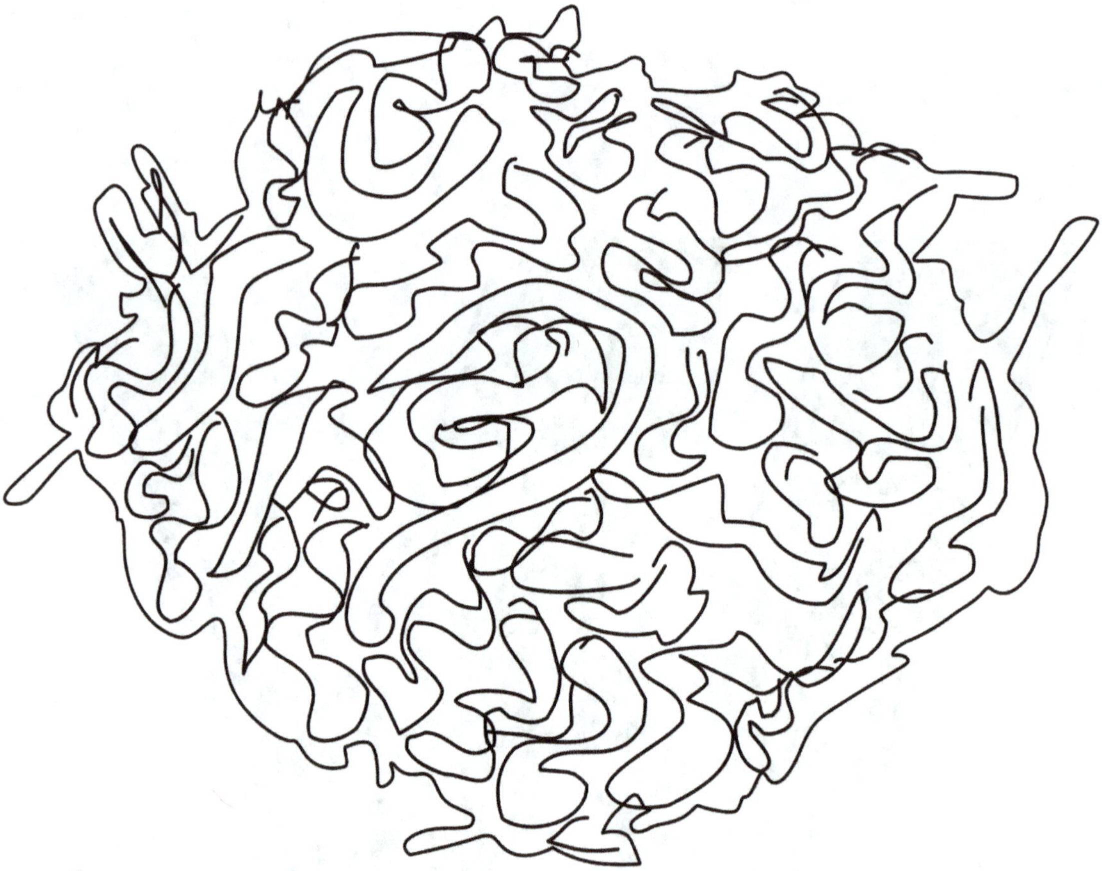

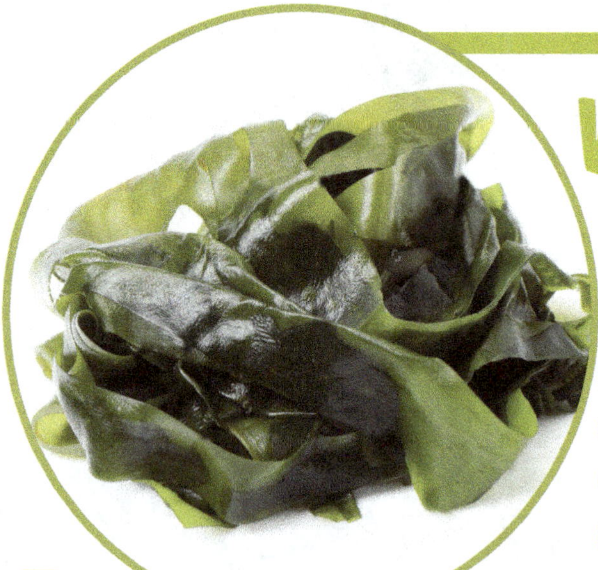

Wakame
(wuh•kaa•mei)

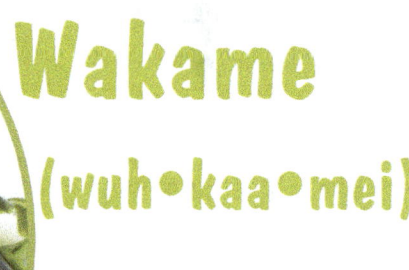

improves brain health, keeps skin clear, increases production of healthy red blood cells, and good source of fatty acids

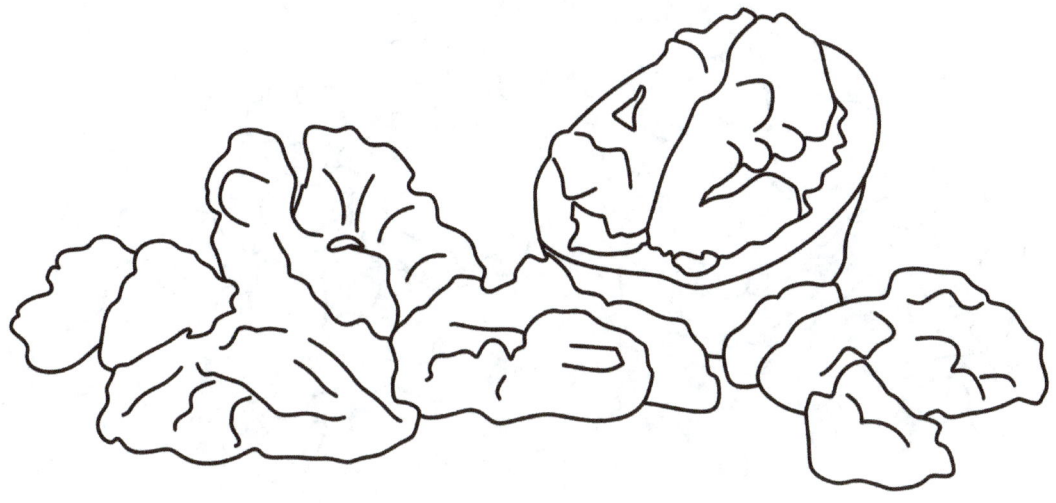

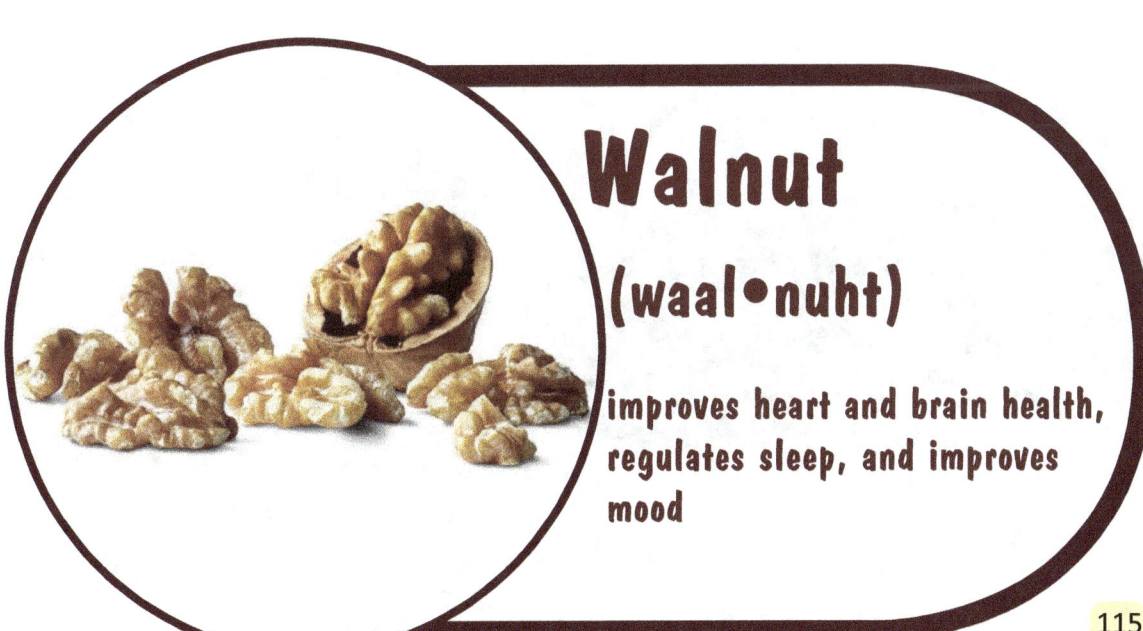

Walnut
(waal•nuht)

improves heart and brain health, regulates sleep, and improves mood

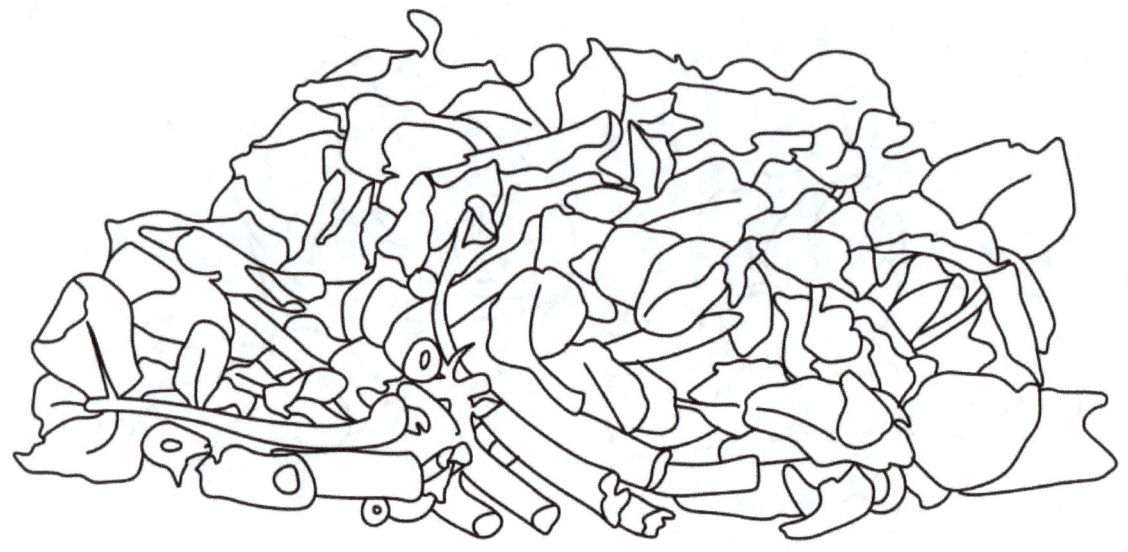

Watercress
(waa•tr•kres)

improves nutrient absoprtion, removes mucus in the body, and fights against infections and viruses

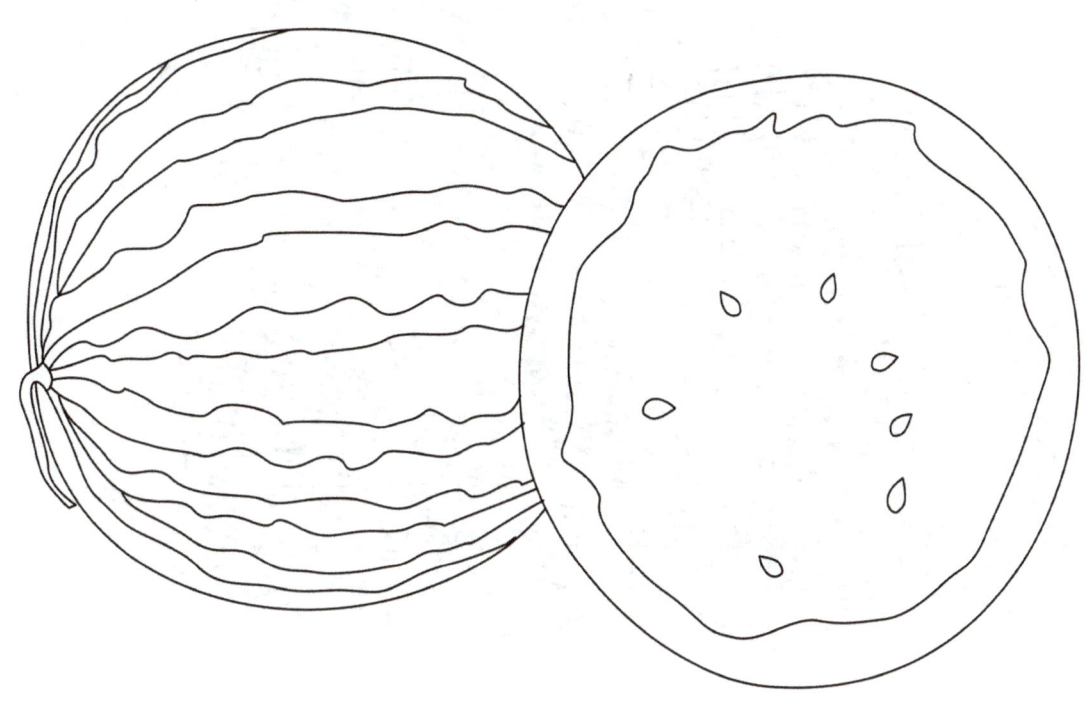

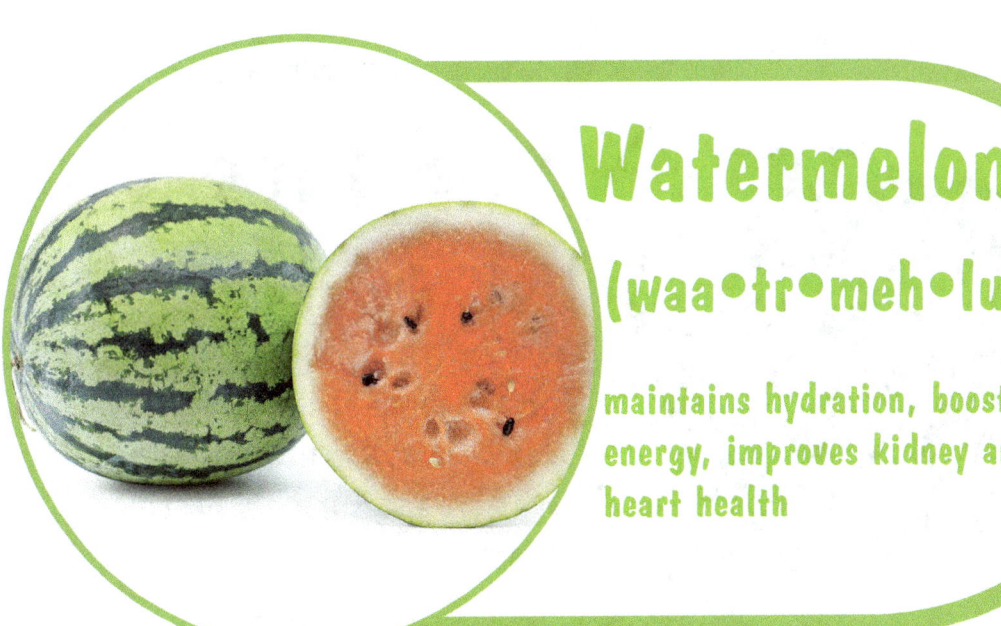

Watermelon
(waa•tr•meh•luhn)

maintains hydration, boosts energy, improves kidney and heart health

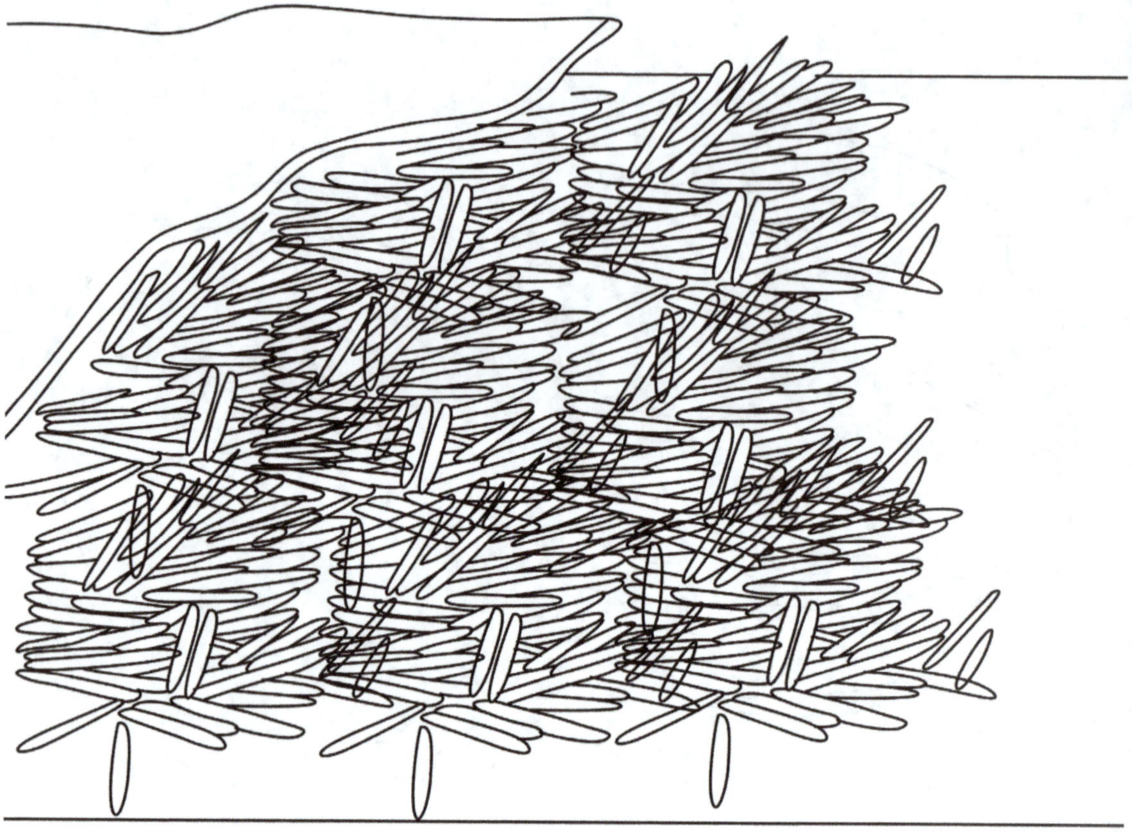

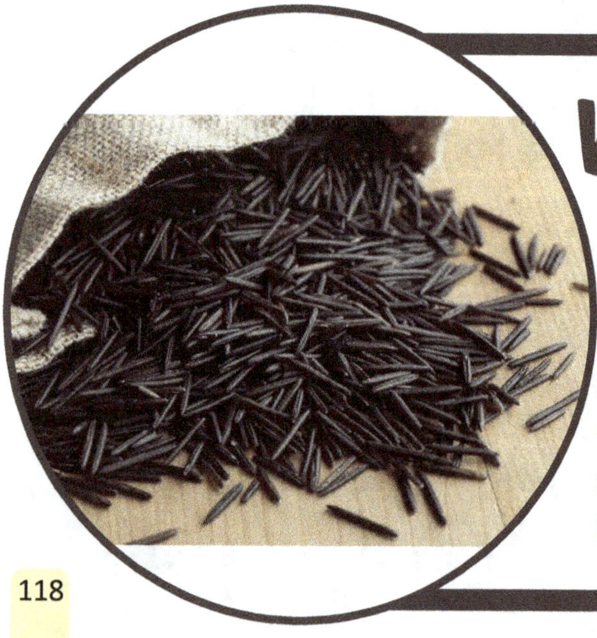

Wild Rice
(waild rais)

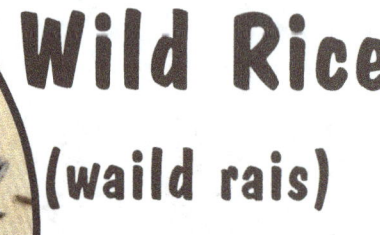

great source of iron, repairs damaged cells, boosts immune system, and supports healthy bones

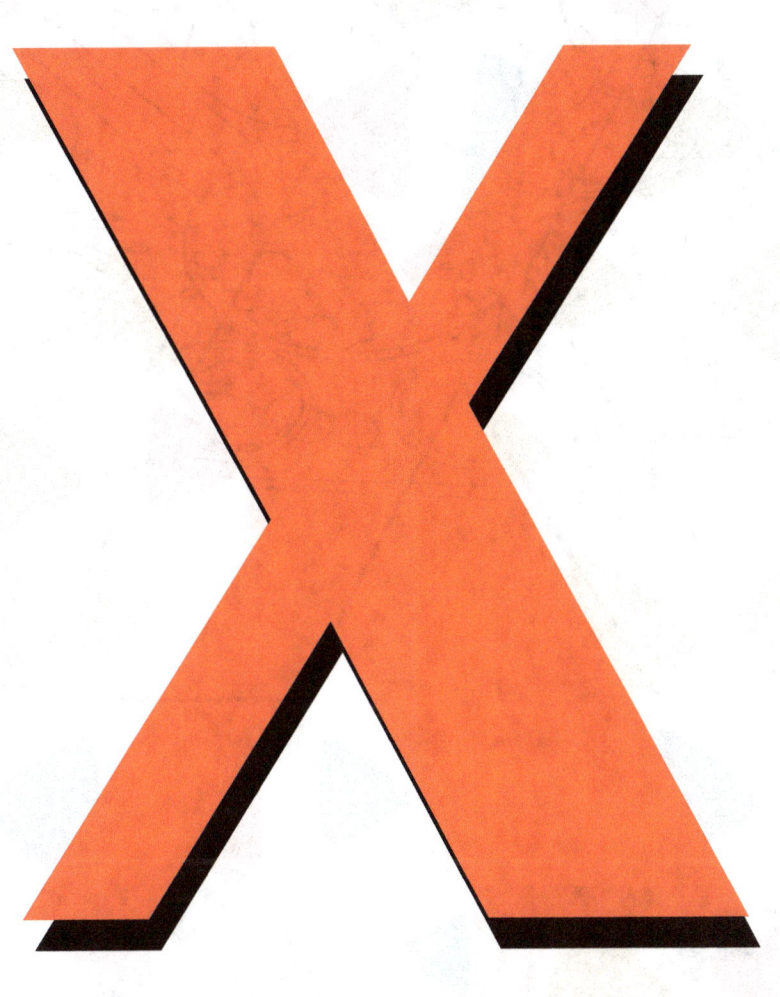

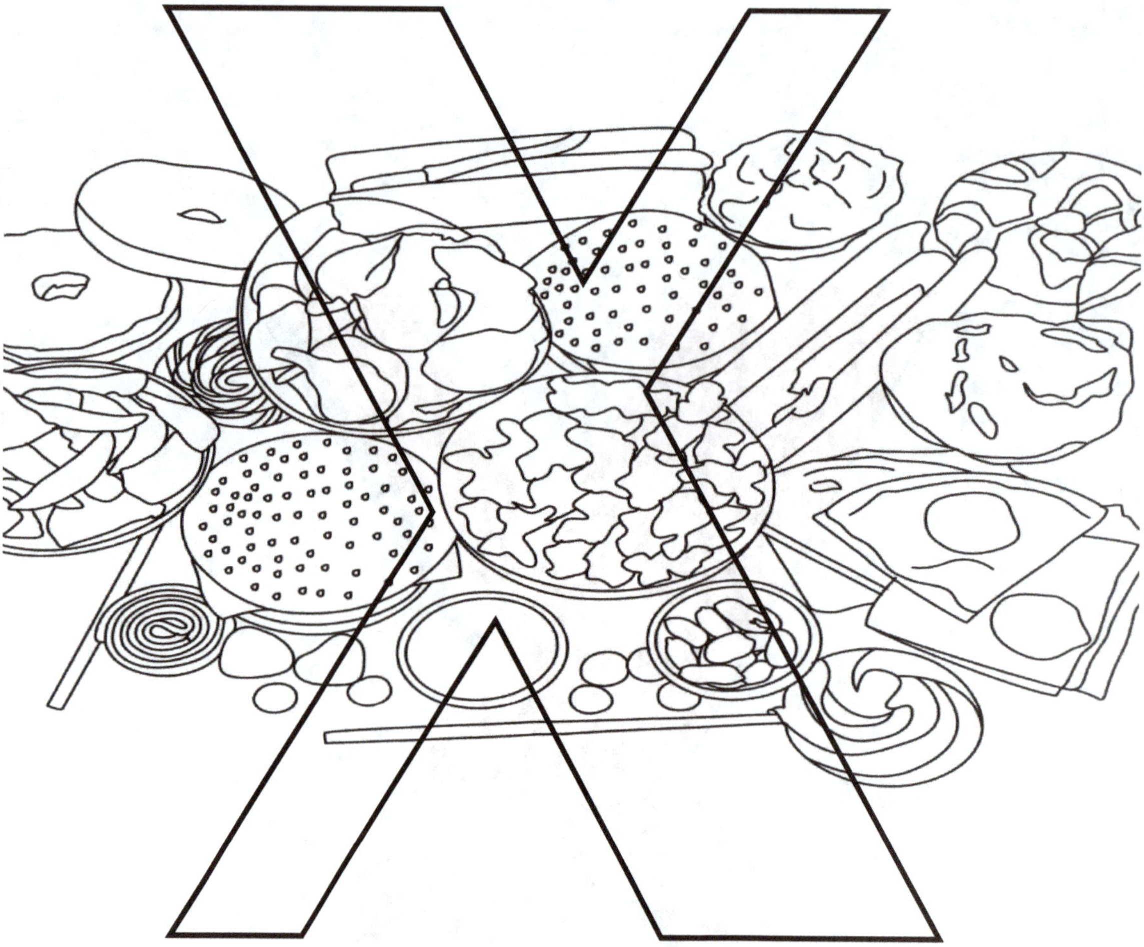

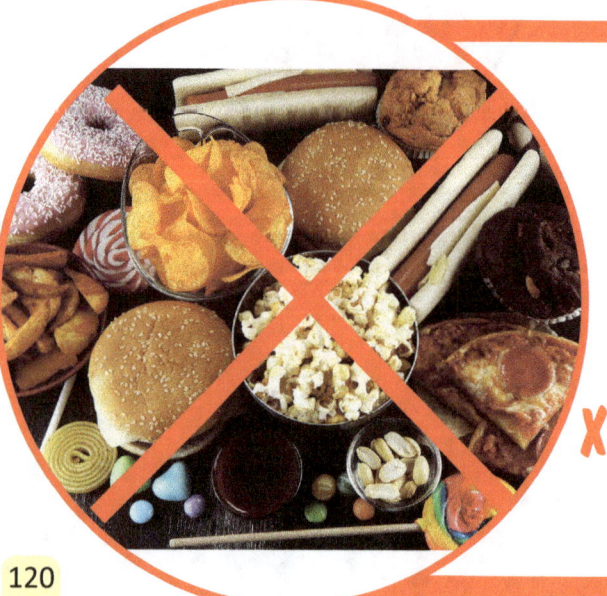

X Soda X
X Dairy X
X Animal Flesh X
X Junk Foods X
X Artificial Sugars X
X Fast Foods X

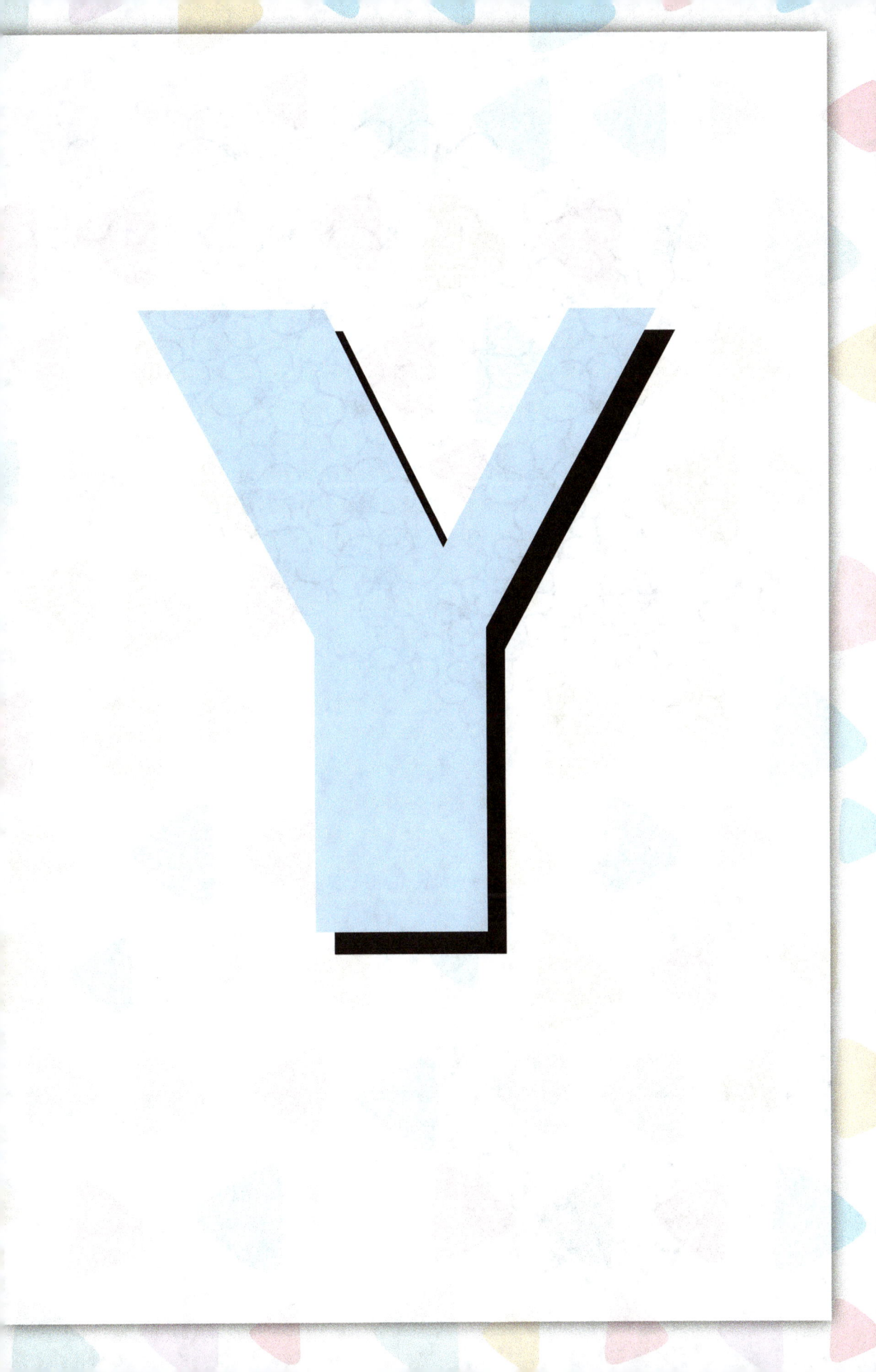

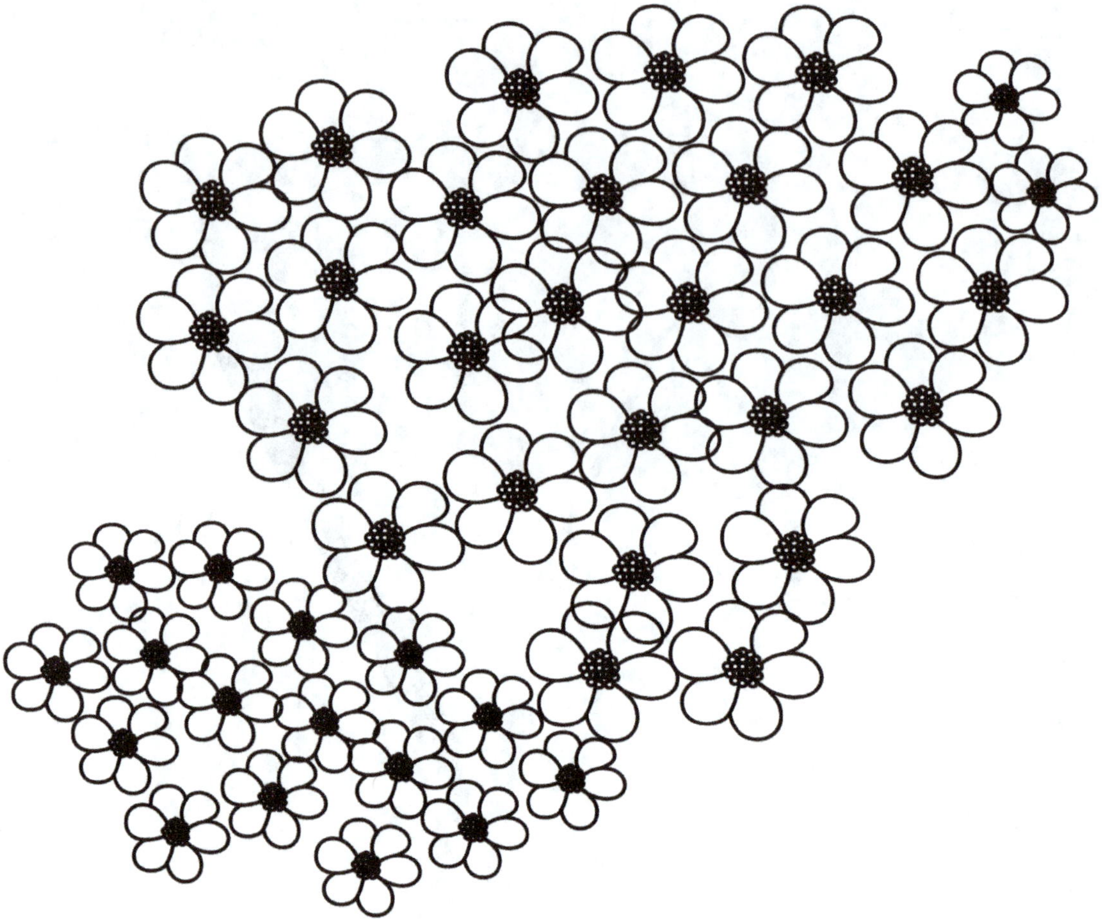

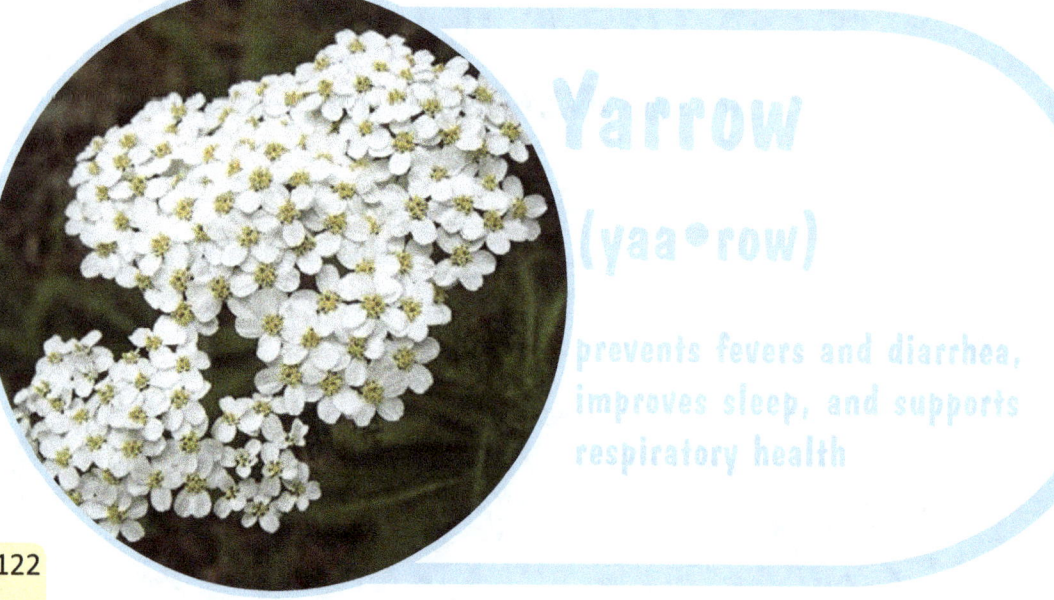

Yarrow
(yaa•row)

prevents fevers and diarrhea, improves sleep, and supports respiratory health

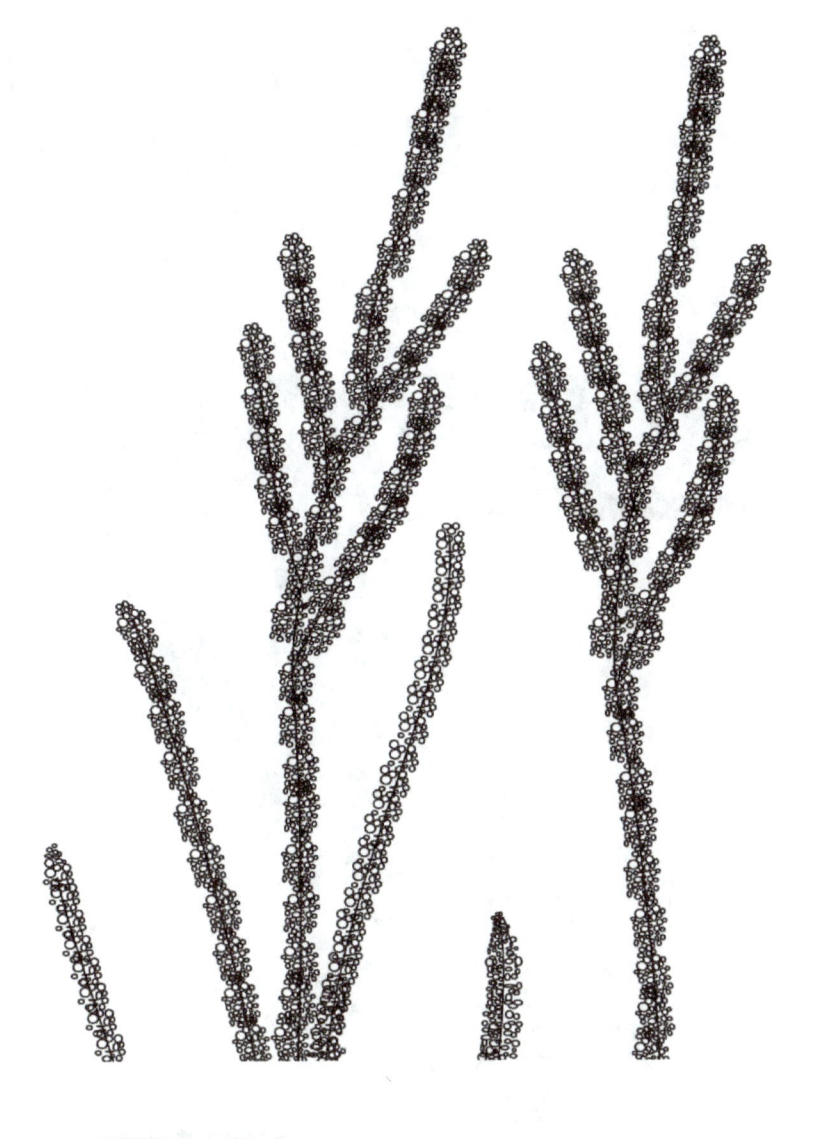

Yellow Dock
(yeh•low daak)

treats diarrhea and stomach aches, good source of iron, and improves digestion

Z

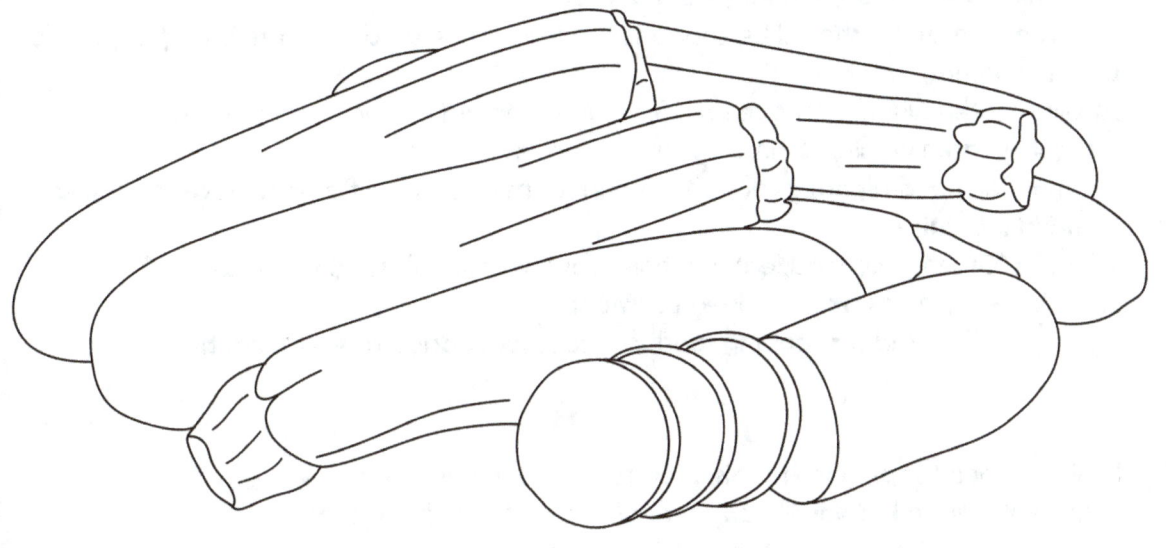

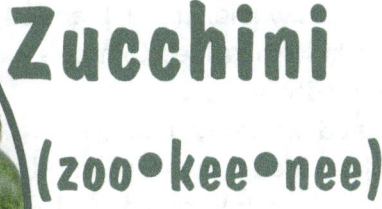

Zucchini
(zoo•kee•nee)

keeps the body hydrated, reduces symptoms of asthma, protects the nerves, and supports healthy eyesight

How To Use Each Item Listed In This Book:

A

Achiote – commonly made into a powder to be used as garnish or added topping
Agave (Nectar) – used as syrup substitute; natural sweetener; added to juices and smoothies; used as topping for grains and/or fruit
Amaranth (grain) – should be cooked like rice; can be used to make bread or powder used for baking
Apple – eaten whole (remove seeds); added/blended to smoothies or juiced
Apricot – eaten whole; commonly found as a dried fruit
Arame (Seaweed/algae) - cooked; used in soups and stews; flakes used as seasoning; blended into juice
Arugula (Greens)- cooked; eaten whole (raw or cooked); used in salads
Avocado – eaten as a side; added to smoothies
Avocado Oil – used for cooking foods on stovetop; added to salads lightly

B

Basil – added topping for meals; used for tea; blended
Bay Leaf – added to slow-cooked meals; used sparingly for tea
Bitter Melon – cut and eaten in small amounts; can be juiced or blended with other fruits
Blackberries – eaten whole; blended
Blueberries – eaten whole; blended
Brazil Nuts – eaten whole; blended; soak overnight and blended to make Brazil Nut Milk
Burdock (Root) – used as tea (sparingly for younger children); can be applied to skin directly in small amounts to help heal cuts, bruises, and scrapes
Burro Bananas – eaten whole; blended; mashed

C

Cantaloupe – eaten whole; juiced, blended
Cayenne – used in salsa; added to meals for added spice; often used in powder form to add to cooked meals
Chamomile – used primarily as a tea
Chayote – cooked; fried; stewed; mashed; roasted
Cherries – eaten whole; juiced; blended
Cilantro – added to salads, soups or stews; blended or juiced
Cloves – commonly grounded up and added to baked desserts; can be sucked on to relieve tooth and gum pains; used as garnish
Coconut – inside eaten; shredded; used as garnish; blended into dip/spread; made into dairy-free "cheese"; drink water from it
Coconut Oil – used on skin, nails, and hair, used for heavy metal pulling ("oil pulling"); added to tea minimally
Cucumbers – eaten whole; added to salad; juiced; blended

Currants – eaten whole; used as garnish; blended; added to desserts; made into "jelly"

D

Dandelion (Greens) – eaten whole; used in salads; cooked/steamed; used as tea

Dates – eaten whole (remove seed); blended; made into paste as added sweetener; blended and cooked to make "caramel" substitute

Dill – added to slow-cooked meals; used as a garnish

Dulse (seaweed) – Sprinkle in soups, salads, pasta, stir-fries, dressings, dips, sauces, and breads

E

Elderberry – eaten whole; juiced; blended; made into syrup for coughs or colds; infused into tincture

F

Fennel – eaten whole; added to salads; juiced; used as wraps; grilled; roasted
- Seeds can be crushed up to add to meals, or often used to make tea.

Figs – eaten whole (with skin and seeds if desired); cooked (remove skin and seeds); baked

Fonio (grain) – cooked like rice; made into bread; made into flour for baking

G

Garbanzo (Beans) – cooked/boiled; blended into "hummus"; roast them; add to salad; made into flour for baking

Ginger – used in hot tea; added to slow-cooked meals; juiced; and used as garnish to stir-fry meals

Grapes – eaten whole (with seeds); juiced; blended

Grapeseed Oil – used for cooking; applied directly to skin lightly to moisturize

H

Hemp Seeds – add to smoothies; eaten whole as a snack; soaked and blended to make Hemp Milk

Hemp Seed Oil – applied directly to dry skin; used in hair for conditioning; used to treat acne and eczema

Hijiki (sea vegetable) – mix with rice; lightly cooked; stir-fried with vegetables

I

Izote Flower – boil the flowers; steam; add to soups and stews
- from the Yucca plant; Yucca is acidic and should not be eaten (following alkaline guidelines); the flowers from this plant are helpful

J

Juniper Berry – eaten whole; dried and used in baked desserts; can be juiced and used directly on skin to treat muscle and joint pain

K

Kamut (grain) – cooked like rice; made into bread; made into flour for baking
Kelp (seaweed/algae) – cooked; used in soups and stews; flakes used as seasoning; blended into juice
Key Lime – juiced; added to water; used to clean chemicals and sprays off of produce

L

Lettuce – eaten whole; added to salads; juiced; used as wraps

M

Mango – eaten whole; juiced; blended; seared
Mushrooms – cooked; steamed; added to salads

N

Nopal – sautéed; juiced; used as a tea; added to salads
Nori (seaweed) – added to soups and stews; used as wrap

O

Okra – cooked; fried; used in soups and stews; oven-roasted
Olive – eaten; toss into pasta, rice and quinoa dishes; added to salads
Olive Oil – added to salads; used in sauces
Onion – cooked; sautéed; used in soups and stews; used to make salsa; used as garnish
Orange – eaten whole (remove seeds); juiced; blended
Oregano – used in tea; added as a garnish; juiced and used to clear up dead skin cells

P

Papaya – eaten whole (remove seeds); juiced; blended
Peach – eaten; juiced; blended; grilled
Pear – eaten; juiced; blended
Peppers – cooked; sautéed; used in soups and stews; used in salsa; added to salads
Plum – eaten whole; grilled; made into sauce; used as topping
Prickly Pear – cooked; fried; made into "jelly" and syrup
Prune – eaten whole; juiced
Purslane – eaten raw or cooked; added to salads, juices, smoothies, soups, and stews; seeds can be used in tea

Q

Quinoa (grain) – cooked like rice; made into bread; soaked and blended to make Quinoa Milk.

R

Raisins – eaten whole; made into "syrup"; eaten with nuts; added to approved alkaline grains when making bread
Raspberries – eaten whole; blended; cooked and made into a "jelly"
Rye – cooked like rice; commonly found in bread form

S

Sage – Frying a strong herb like sage mellows its flavor. Fried sage can be crumbled over a dish to heighten flavor at the last moment. Sage can also be used to add to sauces, and breads; used in teas; can be sprinkled onto salads
- Sage leaves are often tied together and burned regularly to cleanse the air in a home, room, or intimate setting ("sage/smudge sticks").

Sea Moss (seaweed/algae) – cooked and made into gel; made into powder; blended; used in tea; used directly on skin, hair, and nails
Sesame Oil – used in stir-fry meals; used in soups and added to salads; Can be mixed with water (about 1-2tbsp) to apply to head for hair and scalp nourishment
Sesame Seeds – commonly sprinkled on top of salads, stir-fries, or soups. Toasting sesame seeds makes them crunchier and can enhance their flavor
Soursop – eaten whole (remove seeds); juiced; blended; leaves used for tea
Spelt (grain) –cooked like rice; made into bread; made into flour for baking
Squash – eaten whole; boiled; used in soups and stews
Strawberry – eaten whole; blended; cooked and made into a "jelly"

T

Tamarind – cooked and soaked to make into juice (remove shells and strings); blended
Tarragon – added to salads and sauces; used as garnish
Teff (grain) –cooked like rice; made into bread; made into flour for baking
Thyme – used in hot or cold tea; used as garnish
Tomatillo – used in salsa; cooked; broiled; fried; added to soups; juiced
Tomato – eaten whole; added as a topping; roasted; added to salads; made into sauce or paste; used in soups and stews
Turnip (Greens) – sautéed; steamed; added to soups and salads

U

Uva Ursi – mostly available in powder or tincture form; used on skin; leaves used for tea
- only leaves are used in herbal medicine preparations

V

Valerian (herb) – used as a tea; commonly made into powders; medicine is used from root to help treat sleep disorders

W

Wakame (sea vegetable) – added in soups, salads, pasta, stir-fries, dressings, dips, sauces, and breads
Walnuts – eaten whole (break shell); mix with fruits or other nuts; soaked overnight and blended to make Walnut Milk
Watercress – eaten whole; added to salads; juiced; used in wraps
Watermelon – eaten whole; blended; juiced
Wild Rice (grain) – cooked; steamed; boiled; mix with beans and vegetables

X

No items listed for letter "X". Use to cross out any foods that do not provide nourishment to the body

Y

Yarrow (herb) – can be applied to the skin to stop bleeding from hemorrhoids; for wounds; in combination with other herbs, yarrow is used in tea form for bloating, intestinal gas (flatulence), mild gastrointestinal (GI) cramping, and other GI complaints
Yellow Dock (herb) – is used for pain and swelling (inflammation) of nasal passages and the respiratory tract, and as a laxative and tonic. Yellow dock is also sometimes used to treat intestinal infections, fungal infections, and for arthritis

Z

Zucchini – sautéed; steamed; added to soups and salads; juiced; blended

Alkaline Alphabet Image Glossary

A – Achiote, Agave Nectar, Amaranth, Apple, Apricot, Arame, Arugula, Avocado, Avocado Oil

Achiote – https://centerofthewebb.ecrater.com/p/32920018/rare-achiote-annatto-bixa-orellana-25
Agave Nectar – https://spicesontheweb.co.uk/organic-blue-agave-syrup-330g/
Amaranth - https://www.healthifyme.com/blog/amaranth-benefits-nutritional-facts-and-recipes/
Apple - https://www.goodhousekeeping.com/health/diet-nutrition/a19500501/apple-nutrition/
Apricot - https://brainfitresorts.com/apricots-a-daily-nutrition-booster/
Arame - https://healthyfusionstore.com/product/arame-seaweed-100g/
Arugula (Wild) – https://specialtyproduce.com/produce/Petite_Arugula_Sylvetta_2621.php
Avocado – https://www.paulinamarket.com/products/avocado
Avocado Oil - https://www.dreamstime.com/avocado-oil-avocado-oil-white-background-image170176836

B – Basil, Bay Leaf, Bitter Melon, Blackberries, Blueberries, Brazil Nuts, Burdock Root, Burro Banana

Basil - https://specialtyproduce.com/produce/TenderGreens_Basil_3645.php
Bay Leaf - https://www.indiamart.com/proddetail/dry-bay-leaves-9672902648.html
Bitter Melon – https://specialtyproduce.com/produce/Bitter_Melon_7662.php
Blackberries - https://specialtyproduce.com/produce/blackberries_102.php
Blueberries - https://specialtyproduce.com/produce/blueberries_103.php
Brazil Nuts - https://nuts.com/nuts/brazilnuts/raw-noshell.html
Burdock Root - https://www.mucusless-diet.com/herbs-and-benefits.html
Burro Banana - https://specialtyproduce.com/produce/burro_bananas_194.php

C – Cantaloupe, Cayenne, Chamomile, Chayote, Cherries, Cilantro, Cloves, Coconut, Coconut Oil, Cucumbers, Currants

Cantaloupe - https://specialtyproduce.com/produce/cantaloupe_melon_788.php
Cayenne - https://specialtyproduce.com/produce/Red_Cayenne_Chile_Peppers_9995.php
Chamomile - https://specialtyproduce.com/produce/Fresh_Chamomile_8324.php
Chayote - https://www.gourmetsleuth.com/articles/detail/chayote
Cherries - https://specialtyproduce.com/produce/cherries/cherries_295.php
Cilantro - https://specialtyproduce.com/produce/micro_cilantro_1064.php
Cloves - https://www.britannica.com/plant/clove
Coconut - https://specialtyproduce.com/produce/coconut/sprouted_17099.php
Coconut Oil – https://spicerackindia.com/product/coconut-oil/
Cucumber - https://specialtyproduce.com/produce/cucumbers/common_385.php
Currants - https://specialtyproduce.com/produce/jostaberries_15154.php

D – Dandelion Greens, Dates, Dill, Dulse

Dandelion greens - https://specialtyproduce.com/produce/Red_Dandelions_3906.php
Dates - https://specialtyproduce.com/produce/dates/medjool_1002.php
Dill - https://www.plantgrower.org/dill.html
Dulse - https://www.thalado.fr/en/food-seaweed-food-seaweed-cooking-food-seaweed-agar-agar-spirulina-cooking-seaweed-cooking-seaweed-seaweed-cooking-xsl-233_291.html

E – Elderberry

Elderberry - https://www.gaia.com/article/gaia-herbal-101-the-powerful-elderberry

F – Fennel, Figs, Fonio

Fennel - https://specialtyproduce.com/produce/fennel_903.php
Figs - https://specialtyproduce.com/produce/figs/greek_18086.php
Fonio - https://abcofagri.com/all-about-fonio/

G – Garbanzo Beans, Ginger, Grapes, Grapeseed Oil

Garbanzo beans - https://www.bakersauthority.com/products/garbanzo-beans-chick-peas
Ginger - https://specialtyproduce.com/produce/Galangal_Root_618.php
Grapes - https://specialtyproduce.com/produce/grapes/muscat/de_hamburg_9314.php
Grapeseed Oil - http://missambivert.com/beauty-uses-grape-seed-oil/

H – Hempseeds, Hemp Seed Oil, Hijiki

Hempseeds - https://mountainroseherbs.com/hemp-seed-hulled
Hempseed Oil - https://drealfmgrenada.com/index.php/2019/06/17/top-evidence-based-magical-health-benefits-of-hemp-oils/
Hijiki - http://www.sandandsuccotash.com/what-is-hijiki-all-about-the-black-seaweed-used-in-macrobiotic-and-healthy-cooking/

I – Izote flower

Izote Flower - https://www.quora.com/Why-is-the-Flor-de-Izote-the-national-flower-of-El-Salvador\

J – Juniper Berry

Juniper Berry - https://ascent-therapies.co.uk/product/juniper-berry-juniperus-communis/

K – Kamut, Kelp, Key Lime

Kamut - https://avvenice.com/en/content/41-kamut

Kelp - https://www.pethealthandnutritioncenter.com/kelp-iodine-for-dogs-and-cats.html
Key Lime - https://www.specialtyproduce.com/produce/Mexican_Key_Limes_875.php

L – Lettuce

Lettuce - https://specialtyproduce.com/produce/lettuce/baby/mix_510.php

M – Mango, Mushroom

Mango - https://specialtyproduce.com/produce/mangoes_2004.php
Mushroom - https://specialtyproduce.com/produce/mushrooms/portobellini_7029.php

N – Nopal, Nori

Nopal - https://www.melissas.com/products/cactus-leaves-nopales
Nori - http://sedimentality.com/nori-seaweed-chips/

O – Okra, Olive, Olive Oil, Onion, Orange, Oregano,

Okra - https://specialtyproduce.com/produce/okra/green_5949.php
Olives - https://www.quimidroga.com/en/2018/08/08/ingredients-and-additives-for-the-production-of-olives/
Olive Oil – https://opelikaobserver.com/olive-oil-v-alzheimers-auburn-conducting-study-on-benefits-of-extra-virgin-olive-oil/
Onion - https://www.savorysimple.net/types-of-onions/
Orange - https://specialtyproduce.com/produce/oranges/oranges_12315.php
Oregano – https://specialtyproduce.com/produce/oregano_310.php

P – Papaya, Peach, Pear, Pepper, Plum, Prickly Pear, Prunes, Purslane

Papaya - https://specialtyproduce.com/produce/papaya/tainung_14013.php
Peach - https://specialtyproduce.com/produce/peaches/peaches_1805.php
Pears - https://specialtyproduce.com/produce/pears/asian/nakh_12599.php
Pepper - https://www.jessicagavin.com/types-of-peppers/
Plums - https://specialtyproduce.com/produce/plums/plums_4244.php
Prickly Pear - https://specialtyproduce.com/produce/Green_Cactus_Pears_326.php
Prunes - https://specialtyproduce.com/produce/Italian_Prune_Plums_7483.php
Purslane - https://specialtyproduce.com/produce/purslane_5234.php

Q - Quinoa

Quinoa - https://www.jessicagavin.com/how-to-cook-quinoa/

R – Raisin, Raspberry, Rye

Raisin - https://nuts.com/driedfruit/raisins/organic.html

Raspberries - https://specialtyproduce.com/produce/berries/raspberry/raspberry_104.php
Rye - https://crankshaftbrewery.co.uk/product/rye-malt-500g/

S – Sage, Sea Moss, Sesame Oil, Sesame Seeds, Soursop, Spelt, Squash, Strawberry

Sage - https://specialtyproduce.com/produce/sage_313.php
Sea Moss - https://divascancook.com/how-to-make-sea-moss-gel-recipe/
Sesame Oil - https://www.exportersindia.com/sattva-organic-oils/organic-sesame-oil-5004967.htm
Sesame Seeds - https://www.indiamart.com/proddetail/white-sesame-seeds-15347393748.html
Soursop - https://specialtyproduce.com/produce/Soursop_11281.php
Spelt - https://www.ecowatch.com/what-is-spelt-and-is-it-healthier-for-me-than-wheat-1882198500.html
Squash - https://specialtyproduce.com/produce/898_squash_18578.php
Strawberry - https://specialtyproduce.com/produce/berries/strawberry/strawberry_87943.php

T – Tarragon, Teff, Thyme, Tomatillo, Tomato, Turnip Greens

Tamarind - https://specialtyproduce.com/produce/tamarind_9171.php
Tarragon - https://specialtyproduce.com/produce/Tarragon_315.php
Teff - https://www.britannica.com/plant/teff
Thyme - https://specialtyproduce.com/produce/tomatillos_224.php
Tomatillo - https://specialtyproduce.com/produce/tomatillos_224.php
Tomatoes - https://specialtyproduce.com/produce/Red_Cherry_Tomatoes_5363.php
Turnip Greens - https://specialtyproduce.com/produce/Turnip_Leaves_18485.php

U – Uva Ursi

Uva Ursi - https://www.indiamart.com/proddetail/bearberry-extract-20241820173.html

V - Valerian

Valerian - https://www.superseeds.com/products/valerian

W – Wakame, Walnut, Watercress, Watermelon, Wild Rice

Wakame - Wakame - https://www.amazon.com/Chuka-Wakame-Seasoned-Sesame-Seaweed/dp/B00WA3BFP4
Walnut – https://walnuts.org/food-professionals/why-walnuts/
Watercress - https://specialtyproduce.com/produce/watercress_526.php
Watermelon - https://specialtyproduce.com/produce/watermelon_17918.php
Wild Rice - https://www.exportersindia.com/netro-import-and-export-group-pty-ltd/canadian-organic-wild-rice-4665287.htm

X – cross out all unhealthy items

X - https://www.eatthis.com/gave-up-sugar-caffeine-fried-food-red-meat-alcohol-one-month/

Y – Yarrow, Yellow Dock

Yarrow - https://thefewellhomestead.com/medicinal-uses-for-yarrow-the-homestead-herb/
Yellow Dock - http://medicinalherbinfo.org/000Herbs2016/1herbs/yellow-dock/

Z - Zucchini

Zucchini - https://specialtyproduce.com/produce/green_zucchini_squash_1243.php

Other Works By Authors

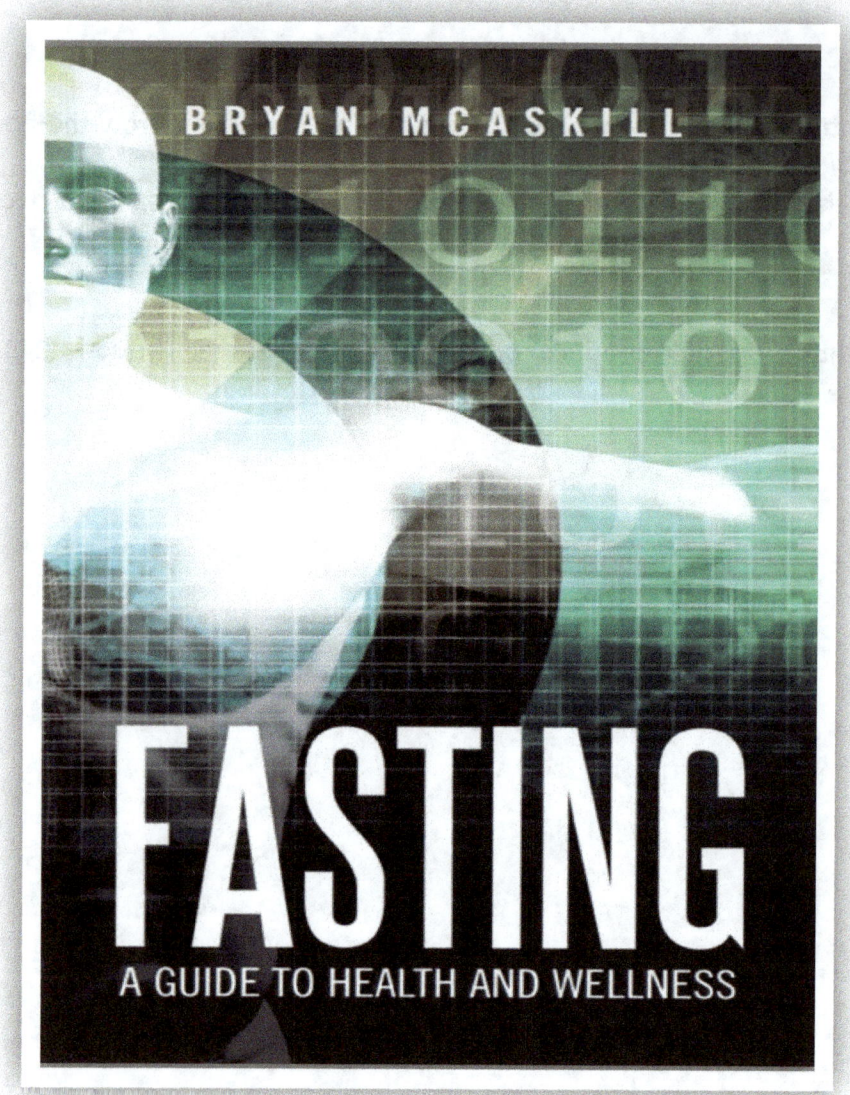

Available on Balboa Press
https://www.balboapress.com/en/bookstore/bookdetails/820758-fasting

Also Available on Amazon
https://www.amazon.com/Fasting-Health-Wellness-Bryan-Mcaskill/dp/1982256796

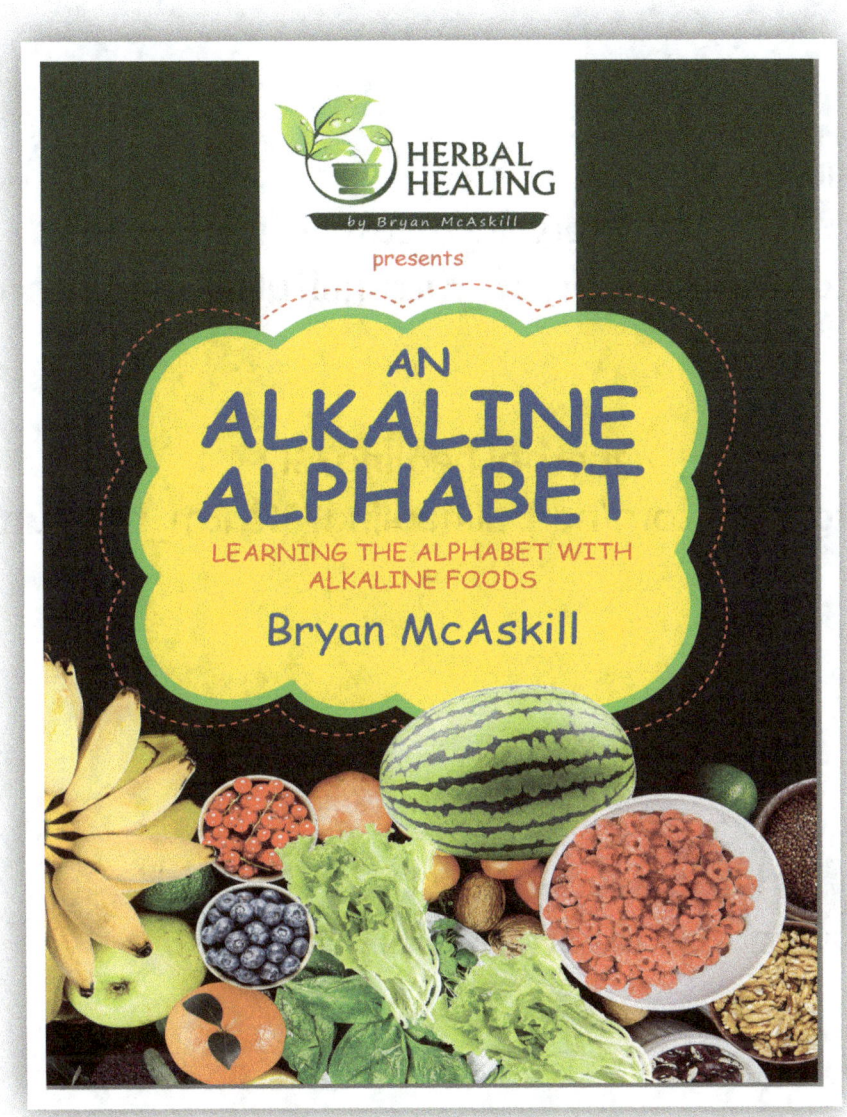

Available on Amazon
https://www.amazon.com/Alkaline-Alphabet-Learning-Foods/dp/0578924021/ref=sr_1_3?dchild=1&keywords=bryan+m-caskill&qid=1624912868&sr=8-3

Make Sure To Stay Connected By Following On Social Media!

Instagram:

@bryan_mcaskill
https://instagram.com/bryan_mcaskill?utm_medium=copy_link

@herbal.healing781
https://instagram.com/herbal.healing781?utm_medium=-copy_link

Facebook:

Herbal Healing by Bryan McAskill
https://www.facebook.com/herbal.healing781/

Thank you **for your purchase and for reading this book.**
Hope you've enjoyed it!

www.ingramcontent.com/pod-product-compliance
Lightning Source LLC
Chambersburg PA
CBHW051212290426
44109CB00021B/2429